Limits of Scientific Psychiatry:

The Role of Uncertainty in Mental Health

by

John O. Beahrs, M.D.

BRUNNER/MAZEL, *Publishers* • NEW YORK

Original graphics by Bowman Hastie.

The views set forth in this book are the author's own and not those of the Veterans Administration.

Library of Congress Cataloging-in-Publication Data

Beahrs, John O., 1940–
    Limits of scientific psychiatry.

    Bibliography: p. 211
    Includes index.
    1. Psychiatry. 2. Uncertainty. 3. Psychiatry—
Case studies. I. Title. [DNLM: 1. Mental Disorders—
diagnosis—case studies. 2. Psychiatry—case studies.
WM 40 B365L]
RC454.4.B4 1986   616.89   86-11692
ISBN 0-87630-420-X

Copyright © 1986 by John O. Beahrs

Published by
BRUNNER/MAZEL, INC.
19 Union Square
New York, New York 10003

MANUFACTURED IN THE UNITED STATES OF AMERICA

Acknowledgments

Many people have contributed to the ideas presented in this book and/or provided personal support in the process of writing it; space permits acknowledging only a few. First are my many patients throughout the years, who, in their courageous quest for health, have contributed much of the data that have led to this work. Equally essential are my parents, John and Virginia Beahrs, without whom this project could never have occurred; my uncle, Oliver H. Beahrs, Mayo Clinic, who stimulated my interest in scientific medicine at an early age; and my wife, Claudette, for her support, patience, and penetrating critiques. Helen Hall assisted me in preparing the manuscript. Key influences toward developing my theoretical position were Ernest R. Hilgard, Stanford Hypnosis Research Laboratory; Milton H. Erickson; and John G. Watkins, University of Montana; along with the "skeptical" work of Theodore X. Barber. Karl E. Humiston provided additional exposure to several unusual and innovative approaches. Several colleagues have helped by reviewing portions of the manuscript: Roland Atkinson; George L. Engel; George Keepers; George Saslow; and Claudette. Dr. Engel's influence extended from my medical school years, through his presentation of the biopsychosocial model, to his recent critique of my manuscript, the Foreword, and encouragement in my pursuit of the uncertainty principle. Elliott D. Bloom, Professor of Physics, Stanford University, has also assisted me in comparing and contrasting the roots of uncertainty in our respective domains. To these individuals, and to so many more, I owe a debt of gratitude.

February, 1986   J.O.B.

v

Contents

Foreword

When John Beahrs solicited my interest to critically review and perhaps write a foreword for his new book, I could hardly have known on what a mind-stretching journey I was about to embark. I had not read any of his earlier writings, and I did not associate his name with the John Beahrs who had taken his first two years (1962–64) at Rochester. But his letter had an instant appeal to me. In it was the hint that Beahrs felt that broadening of the scientific approach in psychiatry (and medicine) rested not just on adoption of the more inclusive systems (biopsychosocial) paradigm, with its attention to the inseparability (connectedness) of natural systems, but also on acknowledgment of the uncertainty inherent in natural systems, an uncertainty that limits all scientific precision in a fundamental way. On that promise alone I could hardly refuse not at least to look at the manuscript. I was not to be disappointed. Once I had dipped into the volume I could not put it down. A few days later Beahrs had my one sentence response: "Your book is splendid and I would be privileged to write a foreword."

That was to be just the beginning. Since then we have met together (in Rochester) and have had a number of phone conferences. I have read his two earlier books (Beahrs, 1977a, 1982b) and many of his papers, all new to me. Thus has been initiated for me an extended period of rethinking my own understanding of systems and the biopsychosocial model, a process not yet completed even at this writing.

A long missing link has finally begun to fall into place, the uncertainty principle, which, as Beahrs reminds us, "has become the cornerstone of modern science, forcing physicists to abandon the strict, causal determinism of Newton and LaPlace in deference to a reconceptualization in more fuzzy, probabilistic terms."

Quantum theory and the uncertainty principle in fact provide the basis for the conceptual transformation that is at the heart of the paradigm shift leading to the new systems (biopsychosocial) model. Yet, over years, I have never succeeded in comprehending how to relate the quantum uncertainty principle itself to biology, much less to medicine and psychiatry. Indeed, much that I have read suggested, or even claimed, that the principle applied primarily, if not exclusively, to the microdomains of subatomic physics.

But in *Limits of Scientific Psychiatry* Beahrs was to resolve my confusion with almost disarming simplicity, an experience I anticipate readers like myself, unversed in modern physics, will also enjoy. Indeed, as he develops his thesis, it almost acquires the quality of a blinding glimpse of the obvious. In effect, he invites us to view the psychological uncertainty so familiar in our everyday work with our patients, not to mention our daily experience, as fundamentally the same as quantum uncertainty even if not expressible in mathematical terms. For example, the presence in mental content of simultaneous opposites corresponds to the twofold nature of energy as both wave and particle at the quantum level. In both cases, the psychologic and the subatomic, it turns out, precision in one dimension (e.g., wave) can be achieved only at the expense of precision in the other (e.g., particle). Thus, Beahrs points out, the dichotomies that abound in mental life (e.g., voluntary vs. involuntary, conscious vs. unconscious, dependence vs. autonomy) are as inseparable one from the other as are the wave vs. particle aspects of energy. It is not *either/or* wave/particle, as the classicists disputed in the last century, but *both-and* wave/particle at the same time. Similarly, it is not *either* conscious *or* unconscious, voluntary *or* involuntary, but *both* conscious *and* unconscious, voluntary *and* involuntary at the same time, that characterizes mental life.

To achieve this insight for the reader, Beahrs makes skillful use of a wide range of psychological phenomena and case examples. For those unfamiliar with or uninterested in quantum physics this material stands on its own, providing more than adequate grounds to establish uncertainty as an inherent feature of mental life and thereby a finite limit to the scientific precision with which the psychological field can be approached. But more than that, Beahrs's analysis of the roots of uncertainty at the psychological level makes it more than plausible that uncertainty at the quantum level is actually but a special case of a more inclusive uncertainty principle that operates at every level of the systems hierarchy, from the subatomic to the psychological (and beyond). Uncertainty, in this view, is inherent in all systems interactions. Quantum physics' discovery that the behavior of individual particles cannot be fully predicted may, in fact, be seen as corresponding with a broader psychological generalization known since time immemorial; neither can the behavior of any single individual, whether a human or a lower organism, be predicted with any confidence. In light of that homely fact, it should be a matter of astonishment not that uncertainty characterizes mental operations but that it is equally characteristic of elementary particles. Merely that shift in perspective is sobering.

Quantum physics and the uncertainty principle by now should have once and for all put to an end the classical notion of an objective reality "out there," full knowledge of which can be obtained by an uninvolved scientist as though simply observing through a thick glass window. Once the quantum physicist realized that his every act of measurement altered the behavior of what he sought to measure, he was, in fact, demonstrating the uncertainty inherent in systems interactions. But in the process he also discovered that it was not just his instrument (or, more accurately, the photons therof) that introduced uncertainty into his measurements; his mental processing also did, at another level. Physicians and others who work primarily with intact organisms have always known this, but under the influence of scientific orthodoxy they have tried to behave as though it were not so, as something outside of science. It took quantum physicists, working with subatomic particles, to recognize the revolutionary implications of their discovery that the scientist is not separable from the subject of study. With that insight even such classical pillars of objective physical reality as time and space came to be recognized not as objective attributes of the world in which we live, but as modes whereby we try to organize what we know about that world. Remarkably, this critical new insight has hardly as yet had any impact on the rest of science, least of all on the life sciences, including medicine, which cling doggedly to orthodoxy.

By calling attention to the uncertainty inherent in mental operations, Beahrs takes a long step toward breaking this impasse. Once quantum physics had acknowledged the indispensability of mind and conceded its irreducibility to ultimate elementary particles, it also had to recognize the quality "entity" ascribed to phenomena in nature to be like time and space, also a mental construct and not a true representation of natural processes. In nature what are in fact continua, or at least connected, acquire by mental operation sharp boundaries. Beahrs completes the circle quantum physics initiated when he identifies as one root of psychological uncertainty precisely this boundary dilemma, the dichotomizing of a continuum, the when-is-it-A and when-is-it-not-A absurdity.

In taking this step Beahrs demonstrates that it is not only permissible, it is scientifically sound and necessary to examine uncertainty in the psychological realm in its own right. For psychic uncertainty is not in some way a derivative of some property of elemental particles, as classical thinking would have it; it is an emergent property of a higher system with characteristics distinctive for its own level of organization. And nowhere is the capacity for uncertainty, that is, to be unpredictable, more valuable than in psychological functioning itself. After all, a completely determinate mental apparatus, like some preprogrammed robotic machine, would, in fact, be totally inadequate for life's tasks. Mental operations must be open to the unexpected, that is, to the uncertainties inherent in an environment constantly in flux. Indeed, adjustment involves attempting to extract from nature regularities not yet known, that is, to guessing, or to constructing hypotheses as to what might be, a step that can never be anything other than probabilistic. As the biologist Riedl (1984) has observed, effective mental operations involve a mix of complementary processes: inherited programs predictable because they proved effective in assuring species survival in the course of evolution (and incidentally, which provide the basis for what sense of certainty seems natural to men, e.g., the indispensability of air to breath, food to eat, and water to drink); and the capacity for openness to change required to assure survival of the individual in an everchanging environment. Certainty and uncertainty thus constitute an essential complementarity.

Uncertainty at the quantum level had to be discovered. Uncertainty at the psychological level has always been known; it did not have to be discovered. That it has been ignored, neglected, even disdained by scientists must be seen as an artifact of how Western science happened to develop. What began as a very human struggle to gain control over the unpredictability of life by at least establishing what can be counted on, what is predictable, somehow became transformed by scientists into an expectation, a goal, namely to demonstrate a perfectly ordered world, in earlier centuries a testimony to the perfection of God's handiwork. In the process, absolute certainty became the ideal for scientists to aspire to in their scientific work. Anything less than certain, which eventually came to mean anything not measurable, risked classification as "soft," in contrast to "hard" science. It is this illusion of absolute certainty that finally has been challenged, but not yet ended, by quantum physics.

The ending of the illusion is the step Beahrs now invites us to take with him. To accomplish this he first invites us to become reacquainted with what we have always known, but from which our attention has for so long been distracted by the false certainty promulgated by scientific orthodoxy. In Beahrs's skillful hands respect for uncertainty becomes the order of the day. Interest, curiosity, and finally fascination follow quickly as we discover uncertainty to be as powerful a tool for scientific inquiry as had been claimed for certainty by orthodoxy. By forbidding absolute certainty, Beahrs shows us "something akin to certainty becomes reestablished at a new level." Recognition of the complementarity of certainty and uncertainty opens for psychiatry, as well as for all the life sciences, the same door that had been opened for the physical sciences by the discovery of the wave/particle complementarity. The opportunity is provided for a thorough reassessment of the limits (and range) of science. But for psychiatry the task should be easier than it was for physics. Psychiatrists need only order and systematize what they already know; the physicists had to discover it.

This is the challenging journey Beahrs offers the reader. It is worth every step. At least of that I am certain — reasonably certain, that is.

December 31, 1985   George L. Engel, M.D.
                                     Professor Emeritus of Psychiatry
                                     Professor Emeritus of Medicine
                                     University of Rochester
                                     School of Medicine and
                                     Dentistry

Introduction

LIMITS AND UNCERTAINTY

For psychiatry to merit stature as a rigorous scientific discipline, nothing is as imperative as that it recognize, define and delineate its *limits*, beyond which its tools are useless, self-contradictory or simply irrelevant. A first step toward knowing what something is, is to know what it is not. We must ask what these limits are, why they are there, to what extent they can be pushed by new data or new ways of looking at the old, and to what extent they are fundamental. Scientific precision is limited in a most basic way by the intrinsic nature of our discipline's subject matter; therefore, it is essential to be as precise as possible in specifying why it is not possible to be precise. If modes of thinking, categorizing, and acting, long thought to be "scientific," are found not to optimally address the unique complexities and uncertainties of human behavior, then we must take another look at our basic assumptions and seek new ways to conceptualize our data base. The new type of thinking that will emerge is no less scientific, just different.

The central thesis of this book is that the traditional scientific approach to mental health is limited by so many different factors, that were we to limit our professional activity to what is usually considered "scientific," we would sacrifice much if not most of our vast potential to impact the course of human events. Many factors contribute to undermine any attempt at comprehensive scientific understanding. These include diffuse boundaries, inordinately complex causal networks, and simultaneous presence of irreconcilable opposites. Added to these are such uniquely human quirks as differing value priorities, word connotations, perceptual and personality styles, different ways we establish our sense of pride and direction, and the elusive human need to save face. All of these factors contribute a fundamental quality of uncertainty that no amount of new data can mitigate. Their common expression is an uncertainty principle, an inverse relationship between precision and reliability of our psychological constructs so that the more rigorously and precisely we try to define our understandings, the more likely it is that some oppositional datum will emerge to render our original formulations absurd.

This is not to debunk the validity or value of a rigorous scientific approach, nor to promote or rationalize undisciplined cultism by removing the grounding that a scientific orthodoxy can provide. By carefully delineating the limits beyond which the traditional search for scientific precision cannot go, I hope to stimulate the emergence of a new way of thinking about our data more effective in handling the many paradoxes, dilemmas, and conundrums that psychiatrists face in their daily practice. Clinical interventions can become more competent and creative as well as protective. By forbidding certainty, something akin to certainty will be reestablished at another level. The fundamental limits do not disappear, nor are they even pushed or extended; they simply work for rather than against us. By better knowing what we are not, we can know better what we are.

Primary causality will be forced to surrender its fundamental character in deference to complex circular networks of interdependent systems at multiple levels of complexity. Instead of seeking to correct one underlying root cause, then, we will search for points of maximally effective intervention or *focal points*. It is often difficult to choose between two or more alternative explanatory models. Either-or thinking, then, often becomes either-*and*, requiring of us more acceptance of ambiguity even at fundamental levels. Truth becomes relative, and is increasingly replaced by utility. The role of certainty is replaced by *presumptions*, such as the "innocent until proven guilty" of criminal law. These presumptions are based in part on value priorities upon which the scientific method cannot encroach. With our ideas of causal mechanism less absolute, such uniquely human attributes as freedom, choice, and responsibility acquire greater importance.

The time is ripe for this type of thinking. Psychiatry in the 1980s is increasingly cognizant of multideterminism, and the importance of complex causal networks extending to and from many diverse systems. The biopsychosocial model of Engel (1980) is widely accepted as the prevailing paradigm. That clinical syndromes may have multiple etiologies and blur into other syndromes without clean boundaries is recognized by the liberal use of the word "atypical" in our nomenclature (American Psychiatric Association, 1980), as well as by the commendable acknowledgment that atypical syndromes are sometimes the more common statistically.

We increasingly recognize that a syndrome such as major depression may be associated with such diverse etiologies as deficiency of catecholamines, endorphins, or neurohormones at key sites in the brain; nutritional deficiency; metabolic derangement, or other medical illness; negative beliefs and other intellectual errors; a history of emotional deprivation, abandonment, or abuse; estrangement from one's "true self"; object loss; burnout; moral transgression as well as excessive moralism; "holding in" as well as losing control of anger and other feelings; religious alienation; and a reflection of disturbances in the family and society at large. Any or all of these can contribute causal input to the final clinical picture, and those that are considered most significant as causes are available for clinical intervention. This kind of awareness is an encouraging harbinger of a new type of thinking that I hope to stimulate and nurture in its inevitable growth.

Despite this encouraging trend, the basic assumptions that dominate the current practice of psychiatry remain rooted in the heritage of classical mechanics that physicists themselves were forced to abandon over a half-century ago. Often hidden or at least unspoken, these assumptions include precise linear causal relationships, "truth" as the final criterion for judging beliefs, and controlled experiment as the only valid way to gather data. Implicit is an unquestioned faith in the potential of science to increase the precision and reliability of its knowledge without limit. For any phenomenon, we tacitly assume that there is one and only one *true* explanation, at least there in principle waiting to be found. Disagreement and divergent explanations are taken to be a result of inadequate knowledge correctible with more scientific research data. A corollary to all of this is the ideal of unifying all of our discipline into a single precise, reliable, and fully comprehensive framework. All of these assumptions must be challenged, along with their behavioral correlates that follow.

In clinical practice we often seek to determine if a distressing symptom's "primary cause" is biological *or* psychosocial, betraying a persistent holdover from the mind-body dualism of Descartes. If symptoms are seen as effects of primary causes, then only if the real cause is modified or eliminated can the symptoms be cured. Interventions not directed toward a root cause are considered palliative at best. When they work, the sometimes impressive therapeutic change is discounted as not real change. Unfortunately, no one agrees about what kind of change is "real." Polarization of biologically and psychosocially oriented psychiatrists, the most prominent of many splits within our profession, achieved wide publicity recently when the 1984 APA meeting scheduled a formal debate on the question of whether or not biological research has rendered psychodynamics obsolete. That such a debate could even be considered, not to mention carried out, illustrates how little the biopsychosocial model has taken hold, and how dichotomous either-or thinking still strongly dominates our field.

Refusal to embrace data that cannot be studied in the laboratory, and is therefore considered unscientific, has led psychiatry to reject potentially valuable input from spiritual, holistic, and ecological sources. Others then seize upon the extruded material, often forming fringe cults that maintain a boundary of mutual antipathy with the scientific establishment to the detriment of each, and depriving themselves of the protective grounding that the establishment can still provide. Scientific psychiatrists and psychologists increasingly abdicate the psychological aspects of our work once felt to constitute our basic identity, the void being taken up by social workers and lay therapists.

None of this inspires confidence in our profession. Not surprisingly, when a large sample of physicians was recently polled to find the prestige value they grant their various specialities, psychiatry was at the bottom of the list. It was more interesting to find neurology on top, a speciality known to be rigorously precise and even esoteric, but able to do comparatively little to help its patients get well. This brought home the extent to which most of the professional world still places the highest prestige value on the unspoken ideal of scientific precision over all else. By tacitly accepting this value judgment, psychiatry has fallen into a trap, since nowhere in all of science is there a greater discrepancy between this ideal and the actual nature of our subject matter. By struggling to become what we are not and never can be, we simply consolidate our position at the bottom, while denying the vast creative potential that our very real attributes hold for us, and even for the rest of science and medicine.

Physics is often put forth as an example of science at its best, to be emulated ever more closely by other disciplines. This is ironic since so far it is the only branch of science to abandon the ideal of scientific precision, having done so irrevocably over a half-century ago due to inherent contradictions similar to those we now face (Teller, 1980). Heisenberg (1927) drew on the essential complementarity between the particle and wave aspects of pure energy to demonstrate the inverse relationship between the possibility of precise measure of position and that of momentum. The more we know of an object's position the less we know of its momentum, and vice versa. Adequate knowledge requires both parameters, however, and is therefore forbidden by the very nature of energy.

The resulting uncertainty principle has become a cornerstone of modern science, forcing physicists to abandon the strict causal determinism of Newton and Laplace in deference to a reconceptualization in less precise, probabilistic terms (Bohr, 1961). Despite grave concerns initially voiced by such towering figures as Einstein (1936), this fundamental limitation on scientific precision has paradoxically liberated us to permit scientific study in areas formerly beyond reach, resulting in such achievements as the unification of chemistry and physics. Psychiatry urgently needs to take these same steps: by defining limits fundamental to our subject matter, freeing us from a rigid scientism to a more flexible multiple-systems-oriented thinking, we will be better able to deal with the data.

In psychiatry as in physics, the cornerstone for reconceptualization is an uncertainty principle. It is not Heisenberg's, since that applies only to understanding of position and momentum at the subatomic level. It is similar, however, both in placing a fundamental limitation on the possibility of complete knowledge of our subject matter, and in requiring a new type of thinking to better deal with this material.

Dichotomies like that between a wave/particle contribute to uncertainty just as in physics, but irreconcilable opposites enter at more than one point and at many levels of complexity. Other factors contribute, such as the need to define our concepts precisely for the sake of clear communication even when their underlying boundaries may be fuzzy in actual fact. Most important is the inordinately complex interrelationship between biological, psychological, and social variables in their virtually infinite interplay. The task of science stands against this complexity, being, as Teller (1980) put it, the "pursuit of simplicity." We attempt to draw out patterns that can be grasped, communicated, and manipulated. But the more precisely we specify such a concept, the more we necessarily leave out other potentially important variables that can return to haunt us.

All of the above factors contribute a fundamental quality to an inverse relationship between the precision (P) of our constructs and their relevance or reliability (R) so that the more precision that is attempted, the more likely that they will be proven inconsistent or absurd, therefore less reliable. This can be formulated in quasi-mathematical form as the uncertainty principle, or $P \times R = C$, where C is a numerical constant whose value remains invariant within any specified system.

The uncertainty principle and its consequences are pervasive, and will be described throughout this volume as they relate to the mental health context. Since reliability can be enhanced by deliberately lessening attempts at precision, we develop a much greater respect for fuzziness than our original scientific bias permitted. As we retreat further from the ideal of strict causality, we search for patterns of relationships, or models, useful within a given context that is necessarily limited. Clinical interventions are directed more toward focal points that, when changed, will lead to other changes occurring in many other areas often quite remote in the biopsychosocial continuum. Truth is increasingly replaced by utility, and the protective role of orthodox systems by "presumptions" shared by large segments of the professional community and society at large.

More significant yet for the overall structure of our profession is that it is no longer possible to attempt to unify mental health into a single comprehensive system that is also precise and reliable. Fragmentation into multiple competing systems is unavoidable, and we are faced with the challenge of making this unique feature of our subject matter work for us, rather than bemoaning what cannot be changed. Why this splitting is necessary can be seen by looking at the uncertainty principle from a slightly different angle.

Looking at any scientific theory as an abstraction, extracting certain recurrent patterns from the vast sea of complex relationships, it is easy to see that almost any theory might have validity or utility within a limited context, but that by the very nature of the abstracting process large amounts of potentially important data will be excluded. While the theory or model fits and is said to be relevant or valid within the context at hand, what is left out may be comparatively trivial to the final outcome. In other cases, however, the excluded material is not trivial, and renders the model invalid. Here, the model is irrelevant and another is needed that includes and excludes different data.

It is not hard to see that the more we attempt to make a model adequate — both precise and reliable within a given area — the fewer number of cases it will adequately describe. Therefore, adequacy is achieved at the expense of the model's scope or domain. Adequacy reflects precision and reliability so that the uncertainty principle can be reformulated as $A \times D = C'$, or overall as a mutually reciprocal interaction between precision, reliability, and domain: $P \times R \times D = C'$, with the value of C' again being invariant within the specified context.

This presents the greatest challenge of all to our overall professional identity: Clear communication requires precise words, constructs, and formulations; basic protection requires that clinical interventions be based on some reliable model in order to be more than haphazard, and the scope of what psychiatry is called upon to help us understand and deal with covers almost the entire domain of human living. But because of the fundamental nature of our subject matter, we are forbidden from ever having knowledge that is precise, reliable, and fully comprehensive all at once. Futile attempts at establishing which model is really true must be replaced by a tolerance for coexisting multiple models, one not reducible to another. Psychiatry inevitably must be divided into multiple models, due to the inherent limitations of each; the task is making it work for us and allowing a certain coherent sense of direction for our profession in the face of this multiplicity.

Fortunately, we can have the best of all worlds if we simply embrace more than one model or psychiatric system, using each one only where relevant. While no adequate system can ever embrace more than a fraction of specific cases, it is equally true that rare is the specific case for which some precise model cannot be applied. If collectively the narrow but precise models can largely encompass the human condition, then having access to each part of the whole allows us the potency of technique and specificity of understanding that each model can provide within its limited domain. Our profession can then enjoy the advantages of specialization or division of labor, which has consistently favored complex organisms throughout the course of natural evolution.

The task becomes that of organization and selection. For there to be any reliable way of selecting which model to call forth for any specific case, there must be some overall "executive" belief system encompassing the multiple models under a less precise but more inclusive umbrella. With our new type of thinking, unification will need to be replaced by coordination and organization. Viewing our profession like a symphony orchestra, we need to establish an effective conductor.

Lack of this comprehensive umbrella underlies at times chaotic infighting in the mental health profession. We are like a disturbed multiple personality (Beahrs, 1982b). Perhaps an approach similar to integrating a multiple personality will work for the mental health profession as well. The roadblocks in each case are similar: there are no established rules of procedure for determining whose claim to the executive role is most legitimate and there may be more than one way that would be satisfactory. The approach inevitably will become pragmatic, and the paramount role of value priorities will be unavoidable.

The role of controlled scientific experiment remains as critical as ever, even with the increasing relativity of truth and causality. With our understanding now being organized into coexisting multiple models, the task of scientific investigation simply shifts in emphasis from being a primary purveyor of an illusory truth to establishing limits. These limits protect us from beliefs that are grossly false or irrelevent and from treatment interventions that are either useless or damaging. Only by establishing where a given model works and where it is irrelevant can psychiatry be protective as well as scientific. And, as before, controlled scientific experiment rules — not as king, since certainty is no longer seen as possible, but more as a "supreme court" by which "border disputes" between competing models are resolved to the best of our profession's ability.

If psychiatry is the first of the life sciences to adequately embrace an uncertainty principle and thereby deal more competently with the multiple complexities, intricacies, and uncertainties in its domain, its role among its sister sciences and its position at the bottom of the list may shift dramatically. For the dilemmas with which it deals are not unique to psychiatry, they are only more blatantly exposed. Multiple causality is increasingly felt as a force to be contended with in internal medicine as well, although with its biological roots it may be able to maintain the illusion of nineteenth century mechanics a few years longer. Uncertainty will catch up with all the biological sciences sooner or later, as their dramatic research advances propel them closer to their own limits of relevance. The basic principle should ultimately apply to all science. If psychiatry has been forced by the greater complexity and fuzziness of its subject matter to master uncertainty and its implications sooner, it may prove fortunate for its prestige value and leadership potential.

ORGANIZATION OF THIS BOOK

The theme of this book is uncertainty and its implications for mental health. (Rigorous derivation of the uncertainty principle in mental health is deferred until the Appendix.) The four roots of uncertainty are developed in the clinical context throughout the book, illustrated with clinical case vignettes followed by discussion of their relevance to both basic theory and clinical practice. They are: 1) boundary problems, which arise when we need to distinguish a construct from what is beyond, when boundaries are blurred in actual fact; 2) complex causality, resulting from our simple working models being taken from a vast sea of complexity, thus necessarily leaving much extraneous information that comes back and renders our models invalid. These are dealt with in the first chapter on the basic concepts of entity and causality; 3) the "untestable intangibles" of the psychological level, which pose the greatest challenge to the psychotherapist. These are introduced in Chapter 3 and elaborated in subsequent chapters; and 4) multiplicity, exemplified by the multiple consciousness and the simultaneous presence of polar opposites discussed in Chapter 5 as well as in *Unity and Multiplicity* (Beahrs, 1982b).

Since all of the concepts in this book are interdependent, it has been very difficult to organize it into linear form, progressing from a beginning to an end. An occasional forward reference has therefore proven unavoidable. The content does conveniently organize itself into four broad categories, however, with two chapters devoted to each theme. Chapters 1 and 2 deal with complex causality, Chapter 2 following up the basic concepts of Chapter 1 with the problems our profession has in fully implementing the biopsychosocial model. It confronts the problems of reductionism and closes with a complex model that illustrates the importance of its three levels — biological, psychological, and social — and clarifies the central importance of focal points.

The next two chapters define the psychological level of subjective awareness, choice, and motivation and the subtle acceptance/nonacceptance dilemmas and vissicitudes of language that make this level so hard to specify with scientific rigor. Chapter 3 introduces these basic concepts, and Chapter 4, on interpersonal control and its problems, illustrates the value of a strategic problem-oriented approach as being more effective and efficient in time and cost as contrasted to the more comprehensive long-term psychotherapies. It closes with a discussion of the importance of face-saving, which sometimes must take precedence over an illusory scientific "truth" if our job remains that of helping patients feel well and function better. Because of the dominating importance of the psychological level — improving our state of well-being — it will be discussed again in the Epilogue, "Faith, Force, and Forgiveness," as it points beyond the limits of scientific psychiatry to the more broad domain of human living.

Chapters 5 and 6 confront the essential multiplicity that so often confronts us even when working at only one of the three broad levels. Chapter 5 develops the concept of co-consciousness at the psychological level, which was the topic of *Unity and Multiplicity*. This concept makes the idea of intrapsychic conflict more tangible and defines many of the problems that psychiatrists address at the psychological level. It also provides a more concrete rationale for the strategic therapies that had been described in the two preceding chapters. In addition, Chapter 5 deals with psychic trauma, which plays the central role in so much of psychopathology, and where multiple consciousness becomes problematic.

Chapter 6 jumps to the social level and deals with the dysfunctional splitting within our profession. It illustrates the problem of cults that exist on our fringe, and the split between this fringe and the orthodoxy that prevents the information exchange that our profession so sorely needs. The phenomenon of cultism is compared to creative innovation, leading to the disquieting but inescapable conclusion that it is often impossible to tell one from the other. Chapter 6 closes with suggested criteria for employing an unorthodox treatment modality, in a way that encourages creative innovation while providing professional grounding.

The last two chapters attempt to illustrate the limits of the pure scientific method in psychiatry and recognize the need to work with many different theoretical and therapeutic systems that cannot be reduced to one another, and that may even appear contradictory. Chapter 7 defines the scientifc method as a complex integrated method using all levels of cognitive and intellectual function from the creative hunch through systematic observation, formulation of hypotheses, and controlled experiment. It emphasizes the importance of working with material that is not testable but that appears again and again in our work. If we reject it as "unscientific," we unnecessarily narrow our profession's domain and limit our own usefulness.

Chapter 8 develops the process of differential therapeutics, attempting to make tangible the new type of multiple-systems thinking that this volume intends to bring to life. Since the profession cannot be unified into a single comprehensive system that is both precise and reliable, multiple models must remain our profession's substrate. Which model best fits a patient's needs should be amended to his diagnosis as an Axis VI. I propose to define the psychiatrist's job more clearly as the *executive* role within the broader mental health profession. It is too much to expect that the psychiatrist become an expert practitioner of every modality known, but his broad multidisciplinary education should best expose him to their essential features, including when each model is most effective, when not, and what types of problematic side effects and complications most often accompany their use.

The orchestra conductor is the psychiatrist, and the orchestra sections and their individual members are the particular broad areas of psychiatric treatment and their many submodalities. Given a new clinical or theoretical problem, the psychiatrist's job is to know which orchestra members to call forth. If this is a model on which he is expert, he will continue as the primary therapist. If not, he may refer to other experts, but should often retain the coordinating role for which his broad training best qualifies him.

Throughout the volume, I will present a threefold focus: 1) a study of the usually hidden and unspoken assumptions that often determine our behavior with less than optimal effect, bringing them out into the open where they can be reexamined and, if needed, changed; 2) replacement assumptions for those that are inadequate and pathogenic, illustrated with clinical case material, helping the psychiatric therapist to be clearer with his categories and more effective and protective with his interventions; and 3) respectful utilization of the "untestable intangibles"—a person's sense of pride and direction, word connotations in their infinite variability, the need to save face, and the many other "irrational inviolables"—on which most healthy as well as unhealthy human individuals base their lives. Again, to reformulate our scientific assumptions to better accommodate our humanness is the purpose of this volume.

This introduction will close with the presentation of a complicated case history and a discussion of the dilemmas that this case raises, deliberately leaving them unresolved at this point in the text. Mrs. R first came to my attention over ten years ago when I was on call at a psychiatric facility in a small general hospital. To both understand and treat her multiple symptoms and competently help relieve her distress, one rule of conventional medical and psychiatric wisdom after another had to be broken. While no subsequent patient has so blatantly broken so many rules at so many levels while remaining fully treatable, I have found many of the component themes to have recurred again and again in more subtle or limited contexts. In many cases their effect has still determined the course of treatment and the ultimate prognosis. If rules must be broken so often, we need new rules.

MRS. R: A CASE PROTOTYPE

Mrs. R was a 37-year-old white female mother of three, admitted to an acute inpatient psychiatry unit with the chief complaint of "desperation" and a two-week history of increasing auditory and visual hallucinations that she was not willing to discuss with me "because if I do something horrible might happen to my family." She had first seen a psychiatrist for a similar complaint ten years earlier and had been hospitalized several times during the subsequent five years with the diagnosis of either schizophrenia or schizoaffective disorder.

She had been treated with a variety of phenothiazines and haloperidol in a dosage equivalent to approximately 1200 mg chlorpromazine a day with only equivocal results. Worse, treatment with neuroleptics resulted in idiosyncratic allergic reactions including angioneurotic edema and frank pulmonary congestion. "Possible seizure disorder" had also been diagnosed on the basis of several episodes of crying and confusion with subsequent amnesia. She had been placed on dilantin, again with equivocal results. The patient reported having suffered a significant febrile illness as a child, and recent EEG was borderline.

Further complicating her already distressing story were multiple medical complaints that had exasperated all evaluating physicians: musculoskeletal tension including headaches and similar complaints in her back and extremities; and episodic abdominal distress at times resembling an acute abdomen, but often resolving as fast as it occurred. She had been alternately diagnosed as hypothyroid and euthyroid, depending on the bias of her physician at the time. What is known is that T-3 values were often barely low or low normal, T-4s were high normal, and the combined thyroid index or T-7 was always normal. Yet when treated with thyroid, usually T-3 in a total daily dose of 75 mg, she felt better, functioned better, and was able to keep her weight down.

Developmental history revealed multiple shamings and abandonments, episodic physical abuse, and sexual abuse at least to the extent of being forced to watch others engaged in deviant sexual behavior. She nonetheless valued her family quite highly. Family history revealed diabetes and a somewhat atypical mental illness on the mother's side of the family, but was otherwise noncontributory. Physical examination revealed a moderately obese white female in no physical distress, and otherwise within normal limits. Laboratory work confirmed the borderline low normal T-3, high normal T-4, and normal T-7.

On mental status Mrs. R was cognitively intact but showed extreme affective lability. There were sudden changes between a relatively coherent presentation and frank loosening of associations. She believed that perhaps others could control her mind, and she suffered from morbid obsessive fantasies that were clearly of delusional proportions. Sometimes she suddenly became angry, petulant, and demanding, and at other times fearful, or even tearful as if going through a bitter grief process. Diagnostic impression at the first interview was indeed a chronic schizophrenic disorder, albeit atypical, with an acute exacerbation. In view of the horrendous allergic reactions she had suffered to prior neuroleptics, I chose to prescribe thiothixene, a nonphenothiazine antipsychotic she had not yet tried.

The second day put things in an entirely new light. While discussing her painful childhood, she abruptly lost contact with me and the entire current setting, neither seeing nor hearing us but instead talking in a despairing voice with people neither seen nor heard by me or my co-interviewer. She was whimpering and whining much like a small child in a difficult situation. Drawing from my background in hypnosis research, I could see that this patient looked hypnotized, as if she were in an age regression.

Wondering if I could take control of and utilize this process, I simply joined in as if I were a hypnotist who had suggested the regression in the first place. This was easier than I expected. Within twenty minutes I was able to guide her experience through a wide variety of hypnotic phenomena, validate her skill, and bring her into a normal nonhypnotic waking state by a ritualistic counting down method. She was given a suggestion that hypnosis was a valid skill that she could employ and be in full control of. Except for a fleeting one-minute episode several weeks hence, dealt with similarly, the psychotic spontaneous regressions never recurred.

The psychotic behavior and "seizures" that had been so refractory for so many years had been treated by psychological means only, briefly and definitively. Looking upon these simply as spontaneous hypnotic behaviors out of her voluntary control, she was easily able to reassert control over the phenomena, so that *what was once a symptom became a skill*. No further neuroleptic medications nor anticonvulsants were needed during Mrs. R's subsequent treatment.

Although the most blatantly psychotic symptoms had been dealt with in barely more than twenty minutes, this was hardly the end of Mrs. R's treatment. We were left with a primitive histrionic personality disorder with narcissistic and borderline features, best summarized by global immaturity. This was the behavioral substrate from which objectively trivial life events had been interpreted as if major stressors, precipitating extraordinary coping responses that had appeared as a major psychotic disorder.

Ego-building psychotherapy was provided over a period of nearly three years, dealing with issues of separation and abandonment, all-out dependency-autonomy conflicts, and boundary problems. She tended to project responsibility onto the treating physician for what only she could do for herself, and then rebel against this projected control tooth and nail, a classic example of a psychological "game" (Berne,

1964). Marital therapy was undertaken, dealing with these issues in the marital situation. She was often hypnotized and encouraged to use her hypnotic skills to bring to bear on these other problems, always in an ego-building manner, never as a symptom or avoidance. The overall process was toward maturation.

A year and a half into treatment Mrs. R had surgery for a cholecystectomy and a relatively thorough abdominal exploration. Her surgeon told her everything was all right, and scheduled an appointment a week later to discuss in depth his findings with her after she had sufficiently recovered. During this interim she came to my office for an emergency consultation. "Dr. Beahrs, maybe it is irrational. I am obsessed with the idea that I have cancer, and I can't sleep. Please hypnotize me so that I can sleep comfortably and won't have these terrible nightmares." Under hypnosis, she first transported herself to the recovery room, reexperiencing post-surgical pain, and noting a recent visit from a Dr. X whom she and her husband had known socially when he had been stationed overseas in the service. "Why should he be visiting me now? He is the Chairman of Oncology. Why would he see me unless I have cancer?" Perhaps because he was a friend wanting to make a social visit. The patient was asked to look deeper.

After a prolonged loss of contact, she talked in a barely audible voice. She was now in the operating room, opened up under deep anesthesia, recalling detailed casual conversation going on. One male figure, presumably a resident surgeon, kept saying, "Here's another one! Oh no, another one yet!", etc. After much of this another physician frustratedly exclaimed, "What is all this crap!!" The patient could now hear the voice of her anesthesiologist from behind saying, "Dr. X, her blood pressure is down to 90/40; you had better sew her up pretty soon or we are going to lose her right here on the table."

I encouraged Mrs. R to remain in her hypnotic state, and told her that we did not know whether or not those recollections were factually accurate. She knew as well as I that her capacity for imagination was prodigious, but what she reported was certainly possible. If the recollections were accurate, they would admit of more than one explanation. Thus, it was quite reasonable that she would be concerned about cancer. Was she willing to agree to worry as much as she possibly could for twenty minutes each day, allowing herself to sleep naturally at night? Yes, she was, and the insomnia was relieved as of that evening. She was then to validate her recollections with her surgeon at her following appointment, which she did.

The surgeon acknowledged that her recollections were accurate to almost every detail. The "crap" referred to had been a mass of intraabdominal adhesions, suggesting some prior inflammatory process of which he had not been aware. There was no evidence of cancer. The frequent bouts of acute abdominal discomfort for which no cause had been found, and which had even led to a prior diagnosis of Munchausen syndrome, were now clearly shown to have had a physical basis. What that was remains obscure to this day.

The following year the patient was admitted in order to thoroughly assess her reported hypersensitivity to a variety of foods, pollen, and environmental chemicals. Because her symptoms were so severe but diffused and had proven so elusive to medical evaluation, the method of clinical ecology was chosen, per Dickey (1976) and Bell (1982). She tolerated a four-day food fast uneventfully, but on subsequent rotating meals of simple single-test items, she manifested a variety of specific physical and psychological symptoms ranging from itching to tachycardia, and simple dysphoria to dysfunctional rage and hallucinations. The list covered virtually the entire gamut of symptoms that the patient had suffered, most of which had been discounted by the medical community. One reaction was severe enough to require intravenous hydrocortisone, probably due to a chemical preservative inadvertently introduced into a test meal. She was advised to follow a rotation diet similar to that recommended by clinical ecologists. Since she agreed that she was not to tune out from society as a whole, she would not be able to totally avoid noxious contacts; thus some episodic reactions would necessarily remain her lot.

The following year, after three years of intensive work on her immature personality disorder, treatment was terminated. The patient experienced remarkably little separation anxiety, even acknowledging that I had occasionally been a "thorn in her side." Due to her many atypical features, I wrote a summary problem list to share as she desired with other physicians. This list included 1) dissociative reactions; 2) general emotional immaturity; 3) psychosomatic disorders, tension headaches, history of Munchausen's (with subsequent physical findings invalidating that diagnosis), and multiple environmental allergies/sensitivities not well understood; 4) thyroid status: alternately diagnosed as hypothyroid and euthyroid, lab values as noted in the presentation. A pathologist had suggested that there might be an in-born error of metabolic conversion of T-3 and T-4 that could manifest with clinical symptoms even in the presence of normal T-7s; continuing treatment with T-3 was advised for this reason, and more importantly, not arguing with results.

In follow-up four years later the patient was doing well, earning a mid-five-figure income managing a fabric shop, contacting me only to request advice concerning how to deal with a difficult family problem.

MRS. R: ISSUES RAISED

The perplexing yet successful case of Mrs. R exemplifies many of the troublesome issues that I will discuss throughout this book, those that I believe warrant a new type of scientific thinking if our profession is to meet the responsibility of adequately conceptualizing and treating its complex multifactorial subject matter. Mrs. R illustrates the dilemmas of traditional diagnosis, short- and long-term treatment, the nature of hypnosis and dissociation, and consciousness under deep anesthesia. No less important are the medical incongruities so evident at surgery and subsequent environmental sensitivity testing. Later I will discuss these issues in depth. For now, I will briefly review them one by one as they apply to Mrs. R.

Mrs. R pushes the limits of traditional psychiatric diagnosis. Both her history, initial course, and presenting mental status would have qualified her for a diagnosis of schizophrenia, chronic undifferentiated type with acute exacerbation; or possibly atypical bipolar disorder. Yet the mechanisms and preferred treatments that these diagnoses imply proved ineffectual and even dangerous to her. An alternative explanation — seeing her in spontaneous hypnotic trances beyond her control — proved sufficient to resolve conclusively her major disorder, with little effort and no side effects.

Her "thyroid disorder" was the mirror image of this incongruity: She clearly did *not* meet criteria for a medical abnormality, but the treatment that such a diagnosis implied proved successful. In few cases have I seen such a clear dissociation between what is "true" according to operational criteria, and what works in the arena of everyday living. A new scientific thinking must be far better able to deal with the latter, as it is the arena where our professional responsibility lies.

The distinction between long- and short-term treatment is another issue raised by the case of Mrs. R. It is evident that it is at least possible in an occasional case to treat a severe psychotic disturbance by psychological means only, not only briefly but definitively. Whether this will prove to be a clinical freak of nature or a comparatively widespread phenomenon must await collective clinical evidence. It should be noted, however, that although the psychotic behavior was relieved almost immediately, here was an individual whose primitive personality disorder still left her disabled in dealing with many facets of her life. For this there were no shortcuts. With increasing pressure from insurance companies and government agencies to produce results and demonstrate cost-effectiveness, it is increasingly incumbent upon us to clarify when short-term treatment is appropriate and when long-term treatment is essential.

Then there is the matter of psychophysiological reactivity. Clear distressing physical symptoms met no known medical parameters with the result that Mrs. R first was written off as a "crock." Only at subsequent laparotomy did she show clear evidence for prior physical insults. Their cause still remains obscure, not fitting known medical syndromes. That they might have been dependent on her state of mind raises the issue of to what extent ego states can be considered as separate entities. Like so many others, Mrs. R reported that she would be intolerant of some agent in one state of mind, but not in others.

Subsequent recall of "unconscious" material experienced in deep anesthesia is not uncommon. Since the material and its associated experience could be recalled after the incident, it must have been conscious at some level. Experienced hypnotherapists generally can cite many similar case reports of their own. Not only does this auger for more caution in operating room conversation, it provides empirical data on the relativity of the word "unconscious"—there is clear conscious awareness even in *chemical* "unconsciousness."

Two aspects of Mrs. R's case clarify the need to indicate when to use unorthodox formulations and modalities. First was the proven value of a radically different formulation of the psychotic disorder as "spontaneous hypnosis," allowing the therapist to utilize techniques well known to hypnotherapists that would render the phenomenon a skill. Second, the environmental sensitivities do not make sense in traditional medical terms but are classic for an alternative medical model proposed by Dickey (1976) and called clinical ecology. Hypnosis and consciousness have been dealt with in depth in *Unity and Multiplicity* (Beahrs, 1982b) and here more briefly in Chapter 5. Clinical ecology and indications for unusual and unorthodox modalities are discussed further in Chapter 6.

To explain Mrs. R's psychotic symptoms by calling them spontaneous hypnosis explains nothing, since we do not understand the nature of hypnosis any more than we truly understand the nature of psychosis or mental functioning in general. Similarly, to explain her multiple medical symptoms by means of proven environmental sensitivities proves nothing since we do not have the slightest idea at this point what underlies those sensitivities. These would be pseudoexplanations, only linking phenomena that need to be explained. This is still of immense value, however, since there is an increasing body of professional experience on how to manipulate these phenomena for the patient's improved health. This leads us to another point for accepting uncertainty: If we wait for better understanding about what we can already easily do now, we might wait indefinitely.

1

Structure and Causality

OVERVIEW

Any significant rethinking of our premises must start with the basics, which are unspoken more often than not. These are the concepts of entity and causality and issues that arise in transferring these to the more complex domain of psychological constructs, states of mind, psychiatric diagnoses, and theoretical frameworks. An *entity* is a form, a pattern of relationships relatively stable over a finite period of time with boundaries separating it from what it is not. Boundaries are relatively discrete but not absolute. With all that exists blurring into a continuum of intermingling forces and counterforces, any entity must ultimately prove to be an abstraction (Beahrs, 1977a) that will have some fuzziness in its boundary definition. For a billiard ball or a chair this would not be a problem, fuzziness occurring only at the atomic level, too trivial for large-scale relevance.

Throughout the field of mental health, however, our very ability to communicate requires labeling, defining, and discussing highly complex and often unmeasurable constructs. They actually do satisfy the definition of entity, but boundaries are so blurred even at the level of common usage that they introduce an element of uncertainty that pervades almost every corner of our professional domain. They underlie the A/Not-A Absurdity (Beahrs, 1982b). Practical exigencies force us to distinguish a concept A from its converse Not-A along what is actually a continuum, with the result that across the boundary two nearly identical situations are treated as if they were opposite, both pragmatic and logical absurdities resulting. A large list of examples will illustrate many paradoxes that plague our attempts at being scientific. Only the first of the four major roots of uncertainty, boundary problems already render the paradigm of Newtonian physics obsolete in dealing with mental health issues.

Causality, a cornerstone of all science, is neither a force nor a substance, but a linguistic device for helping us to organize our understanding of the predictable in nature. Something is considered the cause of something else if it is closely associated with the later event (the effect), and were the cause not to have occurred, neither would the effect. (This is the legal definition used in tort litigation; fuzzy as it is, even classical science can do no better.)

The idea of a progressive chain of causes, or linear causality, is a natural outgrowth of the science of billiards. So is the idea of one and only one true or primary cause. But in mental health we more often find self-perpetuating causal loops or vicious circles that frustrate our tendency to think in linear or primary terms. A causes B and B causes A; there is no linear progression, and attempts to define which cause is more basic or primary prove futile more often than not. This circular causality already requires a different type of thinking; intervention cannot be directed to a cause that remains illusory, but is rather focused on breaking up the destructive pattern. The clinician needs to identify where in the circle he can intervene with maximal impact. This is the *focal point*.

Both the billiard ball and the two-pole vicious circle examples illustrate simple causality, one linear and the other circular. More often in psychiatry we find such an inordinate complexity of causal elements that the idea of a single root cause becomes even more obscure. Simple linear causal elements do exist but they are usually many. Circular causal loops are not only multiple, but apt to be complex and hard to define. They are schematized in Figure 1.1. Light lines represent linear causal elements, curved lines components of circular causal loops. The bold lines represent only those causal elements abstracted by a particular model to explain a patient's problems. When the bold lines are sufficient to make sense of the patient's situation and to predicate effective treatment strategies, the model is relevant as long as the effects of the many excluded elements are comparatively trivial. When they are not, another model is needed. Complex causality, the second fundamental root of uncertainty in mental health science, il-

Figure 1.1. Complex causality

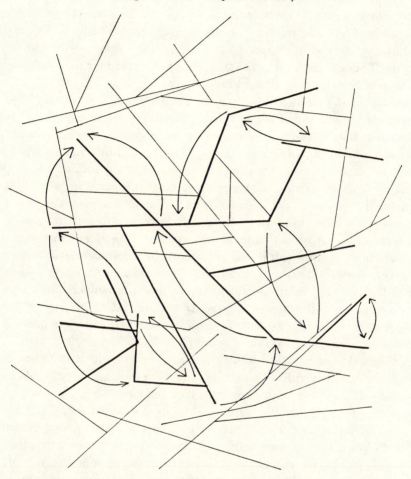

All lines and arrows denote hypothetical causal relationships
Bold lines refer only to those proposed by a specific theoretical system

lustrates why no precisely specified model could be comprehensive (see p. xxiii). The pursuit of simplicity puts even greater emphasis on the importance of focal points.

The remainder of this chapter elaborates on the clinical consequences of the issues of entity and causality, richly illustrated with clinical case material. The greatest emphasis will be on the search for focal points, a task that increasingly replaces the outmoded pursuit of primary cause. Closely correlated to this is the attempt to develop a relatively simple model that fits the patient, providing crisp explanatory formulations and effective treatment methods — the Differential Therapeutic Index (DTI). This sets the stage for material that will recur throughout this discussion.

Accompanying this new type of thinking are several potential hazards to be avoided whenever possible. First is the danger of attributing false causal relationships from random associations found in small numbers of patients. Such *false causality* is common in all science, and the correctives are the same: freedom of debate and, ultimately, the controlled experiment. There are two other types of negative fits, in which a given model appears to fit a clinical case problem and is not grossly false, but where the model leads to problematic consequences. The *irrelevant* fit appears to explain all the salient features of a patient's dilemma, but leaves out some other variable whose importance would render the model trivial. The *defensive* fit, on the other hand, plays into countertherapeutic motivation and supports the status quo rather than the desired change. In both the latter cases it is what is omitted from the model that does the damage: the ever-present emergence of the uncertainty principle.

Clinical illustrations will bring these issues of entity and causality to life as we deal with such problematic but unavoidable concepts as conscious and unconscious, part-selves, and ego states, as well as theoretical constructs like superego, parent, shadow, etc.

This chapter cautions against two philosophical positions supported by the science of billiard balls that have no place in current biopsychosocial psychiatry: "system idolatry," the natural human tendency to see one's own belief system as reality and others' as either false or dangerous — a confusion of beliefs with the reality they are intended to point toward; and the "either-or" syndrome, which denotes the unfortunate tendency to pit one model against another when they would be more effective working together harmoniously like orchestra members, each dominant only within a specific, circumscribed domain. These positions are increasingly being replaced by an acceptance of ambiguity, and of coexisting explanatory models not reducible to one another, each contributing a perspective, but none the whole picture. The trend is toward "either-*and*," which may frighten those who crave certainty, but which will help our profession competently deal with the multiple ambiguities that are there in any case, and move boldly toward a scientific future that not only can fully embrace this ambiguity but reap maximum advantage from it toward the goal of healthy human living.

CASE 1. MYXEDEMA MADNESS

Beulah was a 43-year-old divorced mother of two, admitted to the inpatient psychiatry unit for disorganized psychotic behavior. She had carried a diagnosis of chronic paranoid schizophrenia for twenty years, during which time she spent much of her life confined in the state hospital setting, maintained on neuroleptic medications. The psychotic disorganization occasionally improved, but not the blunted affect, social isolation, and pervasive bizarre quality of her behavior that rendered her virtually nonfunctional as a social human being. Physical examination showed dry skin, puffy face, coarse hair, cold intolerance, bradycardia, slow return of the tendon reflexes, all stigma suggesting a hypothyroid condition. Diagnosis of myxedema was confirmed by laboratory evaluation, the patient was referred to a competent internist, and thyroid replacement gradually increased to a therapeutic level over the course of several months. Within six months the patient showed considerable improvement in thinking and affect. In the one-year follow-up, she was free of all signs of major mental disorder, even without any primary psychiatric intervention. In short, she was *cured*.

Her 24-year-old daughter was now in psychiatric treatment, however, for difficulty with interpersonal relationships and emotional lability. One can only wonder how much of this woman's suffering could have been spared had her mother been given more timely medical intervention.

SIMPLE CAUSALITY (LINEAR)

Cases like Beulah, uncommon but by no means rare, exemplify the ideal toward which the traditional medical model in psychiatry aims: to direct our increasingly refined research tools toward the identification of root causes that can then be eliminated or neutralized through definitive techniques. To overlook an obviously treatable root cause, as happened with Beulah for twenty years, is an unmitigated tragedy;

a psychiatric inquiry always should look first for root causes, even while expecting to find them only infrequently.

However, in actual practice it is rarely that simple, even in a case like Beulah's. While for practical purposes the hypothyroid condition still can be considered a root cause, we can speculate on the earlier causes and complications. Even with a strep throat, usually cured by definitive antibiotic therapy, other potential complications need to be considered. Well known in medical practice is the occasional patient who responds to antibiotic treatment with overgrowth of resistant organisms, leading to complication after complication and occasionally a tragic finale. Thus, even in basic medicine, simple linear causality works only in ideal special cases; it is often approached, but only rarely is it fully achieved.

There is another type of simple causality common in psychiatric practice that fails to yield to linear causal thinking. This is the circular causal loop to be illustrated in the next case example, a prototype of the kind of causality that pervades our professional work at all levels of complexity.

CASE 2. PROBLEMATIC PUNCTUATION

Mrs. B is a middle-aged housewife who came to the consultant psychiatrist's office "for her husband," in a state of desperation. "He is drinking himself to death, and everything I do for him just seems to make matters worse." What did she do for him to try to solve the problem?

> When I remove or hide his bottle that just becomes a game. If I give him logical explanations of the damage he is doing to himself, he just laughs it off. Sometimes I try to be nice to him, but the closer we get the more he drinks. Other times I threaten divorce, but he always comes back to the drinking. I care about him and I don't know what to do.

CIRCULAR CAUSALITY

While we can speculate on multiple biological, psychological, and social causes of the husband's problematic drinking and the enmesh-

ment between him and his wife, at least in principle we can understand the pathology in terms of a simple causal loop, as illustrated in
Figure 1.2. The husband drinks because his wife nags; the wife nags
because her husband drinks. Either way, the causality is obvious to
each participant who responds to the other's actions. In each case it
is probably accurate that change of one spouse's behavior would lead
to appropriate change in the other's behavior. The problem is that all
attempts to define either's behavior as any more basic than the other's
fail, or reduce to absurdity.

The couple can be seen only as a system. The disagreement as to
the "real" cause is not one of fact since both are equally accurate. It
is one of *perspective*, or selective attention/inattention. The husband
sees himself as a responder but not an active agent, and the wife does
likewise. As Watzlawick, Beavin, and Jackson (1967) so appropriately
put it, each suffers from a "punctuation" problem. Each punctuates
the causal loop differently.

In such a case there can be no one single root. However, there is
a corresponding advantage; intervention can occur, in principle, at
any point in the loop. Even though the husband's out-of-control drinking may be considered a more serious presenting problem and the

Figure 1.2. The circular causal loop

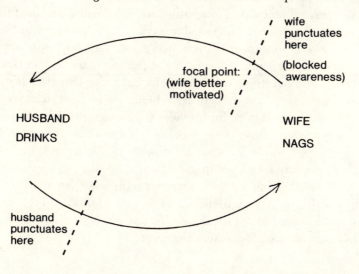

major target of change, he may be resistant to any direct intervention. But *she*, the one who is apparently suffering the most and willing and able to try something different, might be encouraged to strategically modify her own behavior in a way that will render her husband's pathological behavior untenable. Intervention can occur at any point in the causal loop where change is possible — this is the focal point.

While clarity of causality is diffused, flexibility of intervention is expanded almost in proportion. This is the fundamental correlation on which the power of the new type of systems thinking rests and that will be elaborated on at many levels throughout this volume.

CASE 3. BETRAYED

Mr. A is a 35-year-old divorced white male referred for evaluation of a severe depressive episode following dissolution of his marriage a year earlier. He is not actively suicidal, but he has a vague and increasing sense of impending doom. He no longer enjoys his usual pleasures, he has withdrawn from social contacts, and has trouble concentrating to the point that his job is in jeopardy. In addition to losing weight, he goes to bed exhausted only to toss and turn before falling asleep, then awakening in the early morning hours in a cold sweat. He angrily berates himself for "going to pot" but resents any suggestion given by family or friends as an intrusion. He suffers episodic abdominal pain, occasional tension headaches, and vague itching, but physical examination and laboratory work have always failed to identify any source of his distress. He says, "This just isn't me."

A college graduate, he functioned erratically during much of his four years, even spending two nights at the infirmary for "breakdowns," which cleared overnight with rest. He was twice threatened with expulsion for unruly and provocative behavior in class, and was occasionally disciplined both for lateness with assignments and misinterpretation of directions. Despite being attractive and dynamic, Mr. A never enjoyed stable intimate relationships. He established contact easily, but as the relationship grew he became moody, sometimes inappropriately lashing out with a temper outburst, then abasing himself with contrition. His frightened partner would then end the relationship, leaving the patient to resume his pattern with someone else after a brief but intense depressive reaction.

Between relationships were periods of heightened energy and productivity accompanied by an inflated sense of his own importance, loss of sleep, and work binges with impaired judgment. While his "downs" usually followed disappointment in love, the "highs" seemed to just happen. He had occasional memory lapses and experiences of trancelike states, but these episodes always cleared without treatment.

Two years ago the patient married, and it looked like his relationship problems were a thing of the past. However, only weeks later his relationship began to deteriorate. He dreaded that his wife would take advantage of him in many vaguely defined ways, and he would misinterpret and pick at any behavior of hers that he imagined as supporting his fears. His wife felt more and more degraded and used, turning to family and friends for support. A year later, after an explosive outburst sending her to the doctor with bruises, Mrs. A demanded separation. After a brief lull when the patient contritely apologized, she went through divorce proceedings. Mr. A, feeling "betrayed," became increasingly despondent in the year leading to the current evaluation. While earlier depressive episodes rapidly cleared, this one persisted and was accompanied by such impairment in concentration that psychiatric help was made a condition of continued employment.

Mr. A and his younger sister were the products of a stable Protestant family with high achievement expectations. Most family members have done well in love and work, only a few being known to have stormy marriages. His father had been away to war during the patient's early childhood, but had returned unscathed to head his growing family. For Mr. A childhood was "mixed"; no serious problems, but often he had a vague sense of alienation: "I sometimes felt that who I really was didn't count." He could not define that "who I really was." He seemed to get along well with family and peers, but just under the surface was ambivalence and estrangement.

Medical history showed only the usual childhood illnesses and two routine surgeries. Two relatives had been hospitalized for brief stress-related psychotic episodes, several are overweight, a few have ill-defined "allergies," and there is a sprinkling of alcohol abuse. Two relatives had died in their mid-thirties in accidental deaths of which little is known. Family history is otherwise negative and the prevailing attitude toward medical care was avoidance, to "handle it on your own" whenever possible.

On examination the patient described his dysphoric feelings directly and appropriately, along with the anger at himself for not "shaping up." He agreed to a no-suicide contract, but acknowledged both a gnawing dread of impending doom as well as fleeting thoughts that it would be "so nice to go to sleep and never wake up." Most distressing was his sense that he was not in control of either his thoughts, feelings, or actions. He obviously idealized his ex-wife, even while condemning her "betrayal" that he said left him little reason to live. Psychomotor retardation was not present. Speech was vague, but not loose or delusional. He reported rare occasions in the past when under stress he would hear coherent voices that were self-castigating, rigid, and punitive, and on only one or two occasions a voice that was reassuring. Cognitive mental status was entirely clear. The patient was defensive about anything that he felt cast him in a bad light, minimizing and externalizing his problems even while accurately describing their severity. He was reluctant to commit himself to any type of psychiatric treatment, though open-minded to being convinced.

The evaluating physician, Dr. X, representing the best of traditional psychiatry, recognizes the importance of clear diagnosis to organizing treatment strategy. First, pragmatically, he is assured that Mr. A presents no imminent danger of harming himself or others, and feels safe in simply scheduling a follow-up appointment a week later. With the triad of severe depression, insomnia, and absence of acute psychosis, he feels safe also in attempting symptomatic relief with a regular bedtime dose of a sedating antidepressant. Three dimensions of traditional diagnosis must now figure in his deliberations. First are the personality disorders along the narcissistic-borderline continuum. The patient has a history of problems with identity, unstable mood, work, intimate relationships, and impulse control; these qualify him for a diagnosis of borderline personality disorder.

There remains a nagging concern, however, that underneath this surface structure might be underpinnings of a serious functional psychosis like schizophrenia or bipolar affective disorder. Supporting a latent schizophrenic process is episodic social withdrawal and a sense of alienation dating back to childhood, erratic thinking documented time and time again in recent years, the episodic hallucinations, and especially the sense of losing control worsening over the past year. Perhaps he is like a house built on quicksand, waiting to collapse. Affective disorder demands greater consideration, especially with the recurrent mood swings that sometimes seem to just happen. Lack of the deterioration found in schizophrenics is more compatible with mood disorder, as is the fact that most episodes resolve on their own. While affective disorder is now felt to be largely biological in origin and preferred treatment, many such patients have families like Mr. A's where love and approval were contingent upon performance, suggesting other than biological causes. Family history of episodic psychosis also hints at some genetic predisposition for affective disorder. The evidence is insufficient to support either alternative diagnosis, however, and Dr. X chooses simply to postpone judgment.

COMPLEX CAUSALITY

At this point in the narrative I will take leave of Mr. A as a prototype. There is no longer a single Mr. A, but many different individuals, each having the same initial presentation and history as I have so far recounted it. Each is the expression of biological, psychological, and social processes, but each is distinctly different from the others. They merely have the same outward manifestations. As their roots differ, so will their preferred treatments. Dr. X knows that what will work for Mr. A1 will not be optimal for Mr. A2 or A3, but he is already postponing judgment on those alternative possibilities, which fall well into the traditional domain of psychiatry.

Mr. A4, however, suffers from borderline diabetes with hypoglycemia, and gets no help until he joins a faddish holistic mental health society, returning to Dr. X only years later to deal with core personality conflicts that remain. Mr. A5 does poorly there as well, but is fortunate enough to find his place in an alternative medical establishment called clinical ecology (Dickey, 1976). He never resolves personality issues that had initially been obvious to Dr. X, however, and never learns to achieve fully satisfying relationships. Mr. A6 proves to be a covert multiple personality who finds a psychiatrist who can work with him only after years of searching, while Mr. A7 proves to be carrying out a hamartic life script calling for a fatal accident within a year, until this is interrupted by a timely TA script analysis.

This still leaves out the social level. Mr. A8, another borderline with a similar history, makes sense only in his environmental context, where his symptoms have meaning as a "power tactic" (Haley, 1963), achieving passive control where active measures have failed. For him a strategic systems intervention may work wonders, whereas treatment directed to other levels may not work. The list of Mr. A's can be expanded virtually without limit.

Several factors contribute to this state of affairs. Most important is *multideterminism*: the fact that variables at so many biopsychosocial levels can interact in so many different ways to yield the same clinical outcome. A traditional diagnosis or syndrome is more of a common final pathway, what Wender and Klein (1981) refer to as a *phenotype*. In addition is the issue of cause/effect vs. simultaneity.

From the case history described to this point, we are not sure whether Mr. A's mood problems are secondary to a borderline personality structure. If they are, some type of psychotherapy will prove to be the treatment of choice. The reverse might hold, that he has the biological equivalent of a primary bipolar disorder in masked form and that properly treated with lithium, his ego strength might improve to the point that psychotherapy would become irrelevant. Or, less likely, both could be secondary expressions of fundamental thought disorder that would respond only to antipsychotics. Then there are the vague physical symptoms. Are they just expressions of stress, or do they reflect some underlying biological disturbance that they as well as the mental disorder are symptomatic of? Such cases are adequately documented by clinical ecologists, for which routine medical tests would be negative. Clearly what will work in one case will be futile for another.

To further complicate matters, an established modality may act potently at many levels other than those described, and by many different means. Dollard and Miller (1950) argued that psychoanalysis heals more by its behavioral effects than by the resolution of unconscious conflict, and Haley (1963) suggested that its power comes more from passive control dynamics. Psychobiologists recognize that the placebo effect may account for as much as half of the response to psychotropic medication. And even when psychological roots are primary, a timely biological intervention may still prove the turning point, either by breaking up a psychosomatic vicious circle or by permitting the patient a face-saving device. And the therapeutic success of Mesmer's animal magnetism clearly demonstrated how potency of therapeutic results does not necessarily correlate with accuracy of theoretical beliefs (Sheehan & Perry, 1976).

Lazarus (1981) has systematized an approach to treatment planning, intended to simultaneously address all of the levels contributing to the patient's difficulty, claiming that the success rate for this multimodal approach is nearly 75 percent. But a significant number of patients do better not by covering all the bases, but with energy directed to specific target areas or focal points that, when changed, necessarily result in changes occurring in other areas as well, creating beneficient circles to replace the vicious ones. Ericksonian therapy especially attempts to tune into multiple simultaneous psychological levels to find hints for what level might be receptive to such a mushrooming change (Beahrs, 1982a).

Perhaps more than any therapist, Milton Erickson recognized the importance of the intangibles that define a patient's *frame of reference*. A patient's style determined by his use of the spoken language, hidden but still conscious motivations, and matters of personal pride are not just "resistances" to be overcome or worked through, but may be the most important determinants of whether treatment will work, and by what means.

INAPPROPRIATE CAUSALITY

With causal networks so complex and diffused, "truth" carries less weight as the standard by which a theoretical formulation and therapeutic technique is judged, being replaced by the more appropriate question of utility. The greatest risk in the search for focal points is not so much that one will be false, as that it simply will not work as effectively as another might.

False causality is certainly one of several types of error in causal thinking that leads to inappropriate interventions. It happens frequently enough to merit a high level of suspicion in clinical work. Interpreting Myxedema Madness (p. 5) in terms of schizophrenic process was certainly false, and led to the tragic outcome of twenty precious years of a person's life unnecessarily thrown away. Even more common are subtle cases like Atypical Manic (p. 20) in which the clinical course and response to an inappropriate intervention appears to actually validate a causality that may be entirely spurious.

More commonly, an inappropriate intervention is based on causal inference which is not false, but irrelevant. Were the alcoholic husband in Problematic Punctuation (p. 6) to have entered psychoanalysis to discover the cause of his drinking, he might have wasted ten years of his life and squandered away his life savings. The dynamics that would have been identified are certainly not false; they are simply not what is most useful to the situation at hand, the need to break up an escalating marital vicious circle. The dynamics simply would have been irrelevant. Coffee Addict (p. 19) is an equally clear case in which psychodynamics are potentially valid but irrelevant. Here, the simple biological intervention of abstinence was more appropriate.

With Mr. A, the 8 + causal formulations that could potentially explain his illness are probably not either-or, but each might play a role to a varying degree. Whether an element is true, false, relevant, or irrelevant may not even admit of a precise answer. It is more useful to ask the question *to what degree* or *at what level* is a formulation relevant. Where different levels are relevant, at which point to intervene depends on clear delineation of *priorities*, which depends on personal and cultural values as much as on any scientific principle.

Not uncommon is another type of inappropriate causality, which is neither false nor irrelevent, but simply leads to an undesirable outcome. The tragic case of Perfect Primal (p. 45) exemplifies this. The formulation was accurate, that the patient's symptoms arose from difficulty handling anger and grief. And the interventions—emotional discharge and catharsis—were certainly most relevant. But the result was not cure; instead there were increasing regressive dependency and a tragic personality deterioration that need not have happened. The error was not in formal causal thinking, but in the connotation that the treatment modality had for the patient regarding her attitude toward herself. It played into the very heart of her pathology, and could thus be viewed as a defensive fit. Analysis Interminable (p. 76) has similar features. To avoid such mistakes, the many untestable intangibles of life must be discussed within our otherwise scientific framework.

THE SEARCH FOR FOCAL POINTS

A focal point is simply a relatively small part of a person's issues that can be identified, addressed, and modified through an appropriate treatment intervention, and that when changed leads to additional changes in a mushrooming effect in many other areas of a patient's life. The focal point is thus a central cog in a patient's biopsychosocial machinery.

Identifying and modifying a focal point has many advantages over a complex working-through or multimodal intervention. First and foremost is efficiency in time and cost. More is achieved by doing less, especially timely as the need for cost containment becomes ever more pressing on a large social scale. Almost as important is the ability of focal interventions to preserve a patient's autonomy and let him save face. By leaving most areas of his life untouched, they are more likely to preserve and enhance the patient's pride and self-respect, allowing necessary changes framed in terms of his own values, to occur as if by themselves or by the patient's own choice.

The next chapter will continue the discussion of complex causality, presenting the biopsychosocial model and elaborating on its implications.

2

Biopsychosocial
Dilemmas

OVERVIEW

This chapter delineates the biological, psychological, and social levels that contribute to our prevailing biopsychosocial paradigm. It brings this model to life with examples illustrating its relevance to a wide variety of clinical problems. Psychiatry is unique among all scientific disciplines for needing to operate simultaneously at not just one but three broad levels not fully translatable into one another, each level being extraordinarily complex and multilevel in itself. The biopsychosocial model of Engel (1980) is an attempt to integrate these levels without blurring them into one, and is a powerful expression of the new type of multisystems thinking that I hope to facilitate. It also takes a closer look at our profession's self-image; how it perceives itself in relation to science, philosophy, and society at large, as well as how this image affects theoretical beliefs and clinical technique. The theoretical ground for this discussion has already been laid out in Chapter 1; the focus will be on psychiatry in its current social milieu, more clinical and practical in orientation.

The biological level refers to viewing ourselves as living organisms composed of extended matter-energy, identifying and respecting our genetic heritage of anatomic structure, biochemical and physiological processes, and how these can go wrong — as well as made right — by effective interventions. The psychological level refers to subjective conscious experience and its complexities, the "inner" perception of another as it is inferred through verbal and nonverbal communication and empathic awareness of our own. The philosophical dilemmas inherent in developing this level are discussed more thoroughly in the next chapter. The social level respects the fact that no human individual exists or can be understood in isolation, but only in a matrix of external forces including family, peers, and larger social groups. Continual interaction between biopsychological and external influences reinforces the inseparability of the human organism and outside forces. Mandatory to grasping and implementing the biopsychosocial model is recognizing that the three levels are just that—levels—and no more. They are not substances or causes in any sense, and it is meaningless to talk of reducing any two levels to another more basic one. Systems thinking implies that causal levels interact; neither level can be reduced to another, and change at any point in the system will affect the system as a whole (von Bertalanffy, 1968).

Two unspoken assumptions dominate most contemporary clinical practice in contradiction to the basic premise of the biopsychosocial model to which we pay lip service. The first is reductionism, or the attempt to reduce two of the levels to the third, which is presumed to be most basic (Marmor, 1983). The trouble here, besides gross inaccuracy, is that few people agree on which level should be considered most basic. Corollary to reductionism are two equivalent logical errors discussed in Chapter 1: system idolatry and either-or syndrome. The second assumption is a belief that whatever level is considered the most fundamental is the level at which intervention must occur if the resulting change is to be considered "real" change. Both assumptions are natural outgrowths of the type of linear causal thinking of classical mechanics or the science of billiards, and both have unfortunate consequences in the practice of psychiatry.

Besides being less scientific rather than more so, reductionism unnecessarily limits our therapeutic potency far more severely than the inadequacy of current knowledge. Proponents of reductionism can cite convincing data to prove their point for whatever level meets their favor. Psychobiologists cite case after case in which patients have endured decades of futile psychoanalyzing, only to find the psychodynamic conflicts disappear as if by magic when some biochemical abnormality proves amenable to corrective treatment. Psychotherapists point out cases in which clear and modifiable psychological conflicts were ignored or even perpetuated by "pill pushers" until treating patients "like real human beings" led to cure. Some social theorists, such as a few family therapists, virtually ignore the role of the individual, seeing the patient only as a cog in the gears of a complex social machinery. All of the data are convincing, but to maintain any of the reductionist positions requires selective exclusion from awareness of the other two-thirds of the data.

More significant for my overall study is the second pervasive misassumption dominating clinical practice: the belief that definitive treatment must occur only at the level of dominant causality. This is a throwback to the idea that there is one and only one true cause, from which follows out of logical necessity that only if that cause is eliminated will the problem truly be resolved. The inappropriateness of this logic has already been addressed. Further discussion in this chapter consists of examples that illustrate that even when one of the three basic levels appears to dominate in regard to definable causal elements, the focus for most effective treatment may be at some other level and is no less definitive for that fact.

The remainder of this chapter will deal with case examples illustrating where the best level of intervention must necessarily differ from the level of dominant causality if effective change is to be maximal. Two psychophysiological vicious circles common to clinical practice are described. The first is low back pain with muscle spasm. Rather than following the common practice of determining if it is physical or psychological in cause and administering preferred treatment, I will propose a simple causal loop that can be used as an intervention at any point. In some cases a psychological conflict will be the most obvious "cause," but when the pain is effectively relieved by some medical or surgical procedure the grateful patient then proceeds to solve his personal issues on his own. For other patients an organic lesion might be found not treatable by known medical interventions; here therapeutic hypnosis and relaxation therapy might sufficiently relieve aggravating muscle tension so that the natural healing process may occur by itself. Medical hypnosis often works this way, and it is a shame to believe that it should be employed only when biological pathology cannot be found.

A similar but more complex example is the role of nutritional abuse in emotionally hyperreactive patients. The debate over whether or not hypoglycemia is a major cause of mental illness obfuscates the simple fact that what and how we eat influences how we feel, and how we feel influences what and how we eat. A complex causal loop is proposed involving glucose metabolism, conditioning theory, adrenalin secretion, and emotional stress tolerance in reciprocal causal interactions. With this model, multiple interventions could be considered; none would be more definitive than the others, and which is chosen may boil down to such intangible variables as which one best helps the patient save face and ensures cooperation and participation in his own health.

Psychosocial vicious circles are also described, especially the effect of a neurotic patient's symptom on his next of kin or vice versa. On the one hand, a side benefit or secondary gain of a symptom may be to achieve passive control in a family setting where more appropriate methods were futile. On the other hand, the need for passive control may have been the dominant factor rendering some such symptom necessary. Another simple causal loop is proposed, clarifying the fact that it may not be possible to define which level is more fundamental and that, in principle, intervention can occur at either one.

The significance of these illustrations is that they highlight the importance of focal points. If primary causality is either not definable or not treatable, the multiple cause-effect loops may very well permit intervention at spots apparently far removed in the causal chain that will then lead to other changes occurring as if by themselves, perhaps even leading back to the so-called root cause. With the new biopsychosocial model, the idea of definitive cure following elimination of a root cause has gone by the wayside. It has been replaced by something far more precious: the opportunity to choose from many alternatives and the creative flexibility and adaptability that follows. Focal points occupy the same position in the new thinking that primary causality did in the old, while the creative flexibility required for an effective search for focal points is much more true to the complexities of human nature and far more stimulating and rewarding for clinical practice.

CASE 1. COFFEE ADDICT

A 36-year-old male consulted a psychiatrist about a two-year history of increasing anxiety, restlessness, irritability, and insomnia followed in the past two months by increasingly morbid obsessions and compulsions. There were two major life stresses in the year preceding the consultation, one an occupational setback and the other a profound loss in his intimate relationships. Early life history revealed the presence of temperamental and environmental factors, clarifying his especially vulnerable state regarding these recent stresses. Dynamics were nearly obvious, and tentative plans were discussed with the patient for a course of psychotherapy expected to last three to five years, with issues so clear that one could even predict the trouble spots likely to occur in an expected stormy therapeutic relationship.

In the course of routine medical-history taking, however, when he was asked how much coffee he drank, he said three pots a day. Would he be willing to drink three pots a day less? "I can't see how that would make any difference, but no reason I can't try." A week later he returned to the evaluating psychiatrist's office, entirely free of morbid anxiety symptoms and compulsive behavior; in short, for practical purposes he is *cured*. Diagnosis: *hypercaffeinism*.

IRRELEVANT CAUSALITY: BIOLOGY VS. PSYCHOLOGY

If this diagnosis had been missed, three to five years of exploratory psychoanalytic therapy would have been unnecessarily wasted. The causality would not have been false, as the dynamics were, in fact, obvious and even true. Without the heightened anxiety level caused by caffeine, however, the dynamics would not have disrupted this patient's life, they simply would have been his own unique personality structure, the "psychopathology of everyday life . . . " as Freud (1916/1979) so aptly put it. The causality would not have been false, just irrelevant; but just as significant as the failure to accurately diagnose Beulah's hypothyroid condition for twenty years (p. 5).

CASE 2. ATYPICAL MANIC

Clarence was hospitalized for a state of psychotic agitation with loose thinking, grandiose ideation, and insomnia, following a major life stressor two weeks preceding. He revealed himself to be an intense individual with wide mood swings, and a self-assessment known to have wavered between grandiose overevaluation and angry self-castigation. Physical examination was normal and cognitive mental status intact. A diagnosis of bipolar disorder, manic phase, was made; and treatment was undertaken with lithium in a dosage titrated upwards into the therapeutic range. Within several weeks, mood and thinking returned to normal and lithium was continued as maintenance therapy.

Over subsequent months Clarence showed only his normally intense and reactive personality style. Troubled by frequent diuresis and mild tremor, however, and feeling that lithium was doing him no good, he willfully neglected and finally abandoned his lithium regimen. Within a month he was rehospitalized for another psychotic episode, following a strong altercation and separation from a significant other. Lithium treatment was reinstituted, and again within several weeks the psychosis resolved.

FALSE CAUSALITY: BIOLOGY VS. PSYCHOLOGY

Causal thinking in this case seems pretty obvious, at least on the surface. Not only did the psychotic behavior have the clinical characteristics of mania, but the positive response to lithium and subsequent negative response to its self-discontinuation corroborated the hypothesis, an apparent biological confirmation by therapeutic trial. While the intricacies of biochemical causality in affective disorder are not yet clear, the indicators that point in such a direction are well-recognized by the psychiatric profession — bipolar disorder has profound biological roots best modified by lithium and other biological modalities. It would be as unsound to withhold lithium treatment from such a patient as it was to withhold thyroid replacement from Beulah for twenty miserable years.

An alternative explanation might prove equally viable in the case of Clarence, however. A personality disorder of the mixed compulsive-borderline-narcissistic-type might also present with an identical life history of intensity, alternating over- and underevaluation, and mood swings. Such an individual may also have acute psychotic episodes in response to environmental stress, and very often the nature of such an episode will be manic. Such a psychosis will often clear rapidly without medication once a patient is in the secure structured setting of an inpatient psychiatric facility. Whether or not he is on medication, he will be expected to return to his usual personality state after the episode has resolved. He is also likely to have recurrent psychotic episodes under similar stresses in the future whether or not he is taking medication, and it is quite possible that as his thinking loosens he will behave more recklessly. One manifestation of this recklessness might be to discontinue his lithium. In other words, the "obvious" inverse causal relationship between lithium level and manic state may be entirely spurious.

Such false causality is not always problematic, and may underlie many important healing rituals in all cultures at all levels of complexity. It is of major importance, however, when the patient either suffers serious side effects from the inappropriate treatment or when a more appropriate treatment modality is not undertaken that would have been effective.

Such a patient may be reassessed only decades later, when doctors are forced to discontinue lithium because of severe renal impairment, or when psychotic episodes occur despite adequate maintenance. Some such cases will respond dramatically to psychotherapy alone, others will not, and yet others may deteriorate. Clearly much more data are needed, and despite these reservations lithium is usually an appropriate initial treatment for a man such as Clarence. The issues are raised simply to clarify the complexities with which psychiatrists must become increasingly aware if we are to meet our responsibility for more effective, efficient, and protective treatment interventions.

CASE 3. GRANDMA IS DEPRESSED

Mrs. L was a 64-year-old white female admitted to a state hospital for increasingly severe depression of several years duration, now of such severity that she had lost weight, her sleeping was impaired, and she was almost continually wringing her hands in despair about imaginary financial catastrophes and ideas of personal guilt, worthlessness, and hopelessness. Physical examination revealed her to be entirely healthy and cognitive mental status was likewise intact. This patient had been given an adequate trial of several varieties of antidepressant medication titrated upwards to large doses, and had been treated with various psychotherapeutic strategies including insight, awareness, and hypnotic and even strategic paradox, all to no avail.

With considerable effort, the extended family was summoned to the hospital for an information-gathering session, as well as for reviewing the current impasse and planning a mutually agreeable strategy. The family proved to be one of very intense, aggressive, and competitive individuals, with a powerful emotional bonding that was more often manifest by the intensity of disagreements, accusations, counter-accusations, and various colorful interpersonal games. Despite the intense frustrated craving for closeness, the only thing this family had in common was their concern for Grandma. Each was afraid to openly challenge a family myth, for fear this would push Grandma over the edge and precipitate a suicide attempt. Each was afraid to move elsewhere, for fear that Grandma would experience this as abandonment, and wither away and die. The common theme was that everyone had to walk, talk, and think on tiptoes to avoid setting Grandma off.

Within this complex, intense, chaotically disorganized family, who was in control? Grandma. Though the control was passive, forced by the tyranny of her own psychotic depression, and although this control was exerted outside of conscious awareness, Grandma's depression was both a powerful bonding and stabilizing force for the entire family, and served a function that the whole family needed and wanted but to that point was unable to provide for itself. This proved to be the focal point for treatment.

The family was able to accept this formulation without difficulty. Contentiousness turned to cooperativeness, with various family members discussing how they could promote harmony within the family without sacrificing their own unique purposes and gifts. The family was also encouraged to take responsibility for their own actions and allow Grandma to take responsibility for hers. They would say what they felt, trusting our profession to take care of Grandma's psychiatric difficulties. Interestingly, Grandma's depression lifted, and she herself proved to be an intense individual with a sharp, salty wit and a refreshing sense of humor, and was able to actively assume the central role of leadership, which her innate gifts and life experience entitled her to. Had the social axis not been addressed, Mrs. L probably would have remained the hopeless case that she had first appeared to be.

THE PROBLEM OF REDUCTIONISM

Cases such as these, where what clearly appears to be a problem at one level is ultimately solved at another, have a profound effect on the treating physician. After I had shared the cases of Myxedema Madness (p. 5) and Coffee Addict, one psychobiologist validated this impact: "Yes, you see enough cases like this where years of psychotherapy proved to be futile, but antidepressants led to equally impressive results. After a while, you become a believer." This M.D. went on to ventilate his discomfort in the mental health movement, stating his belief that even for personality disorders "we will ultimately find a biological cause we can really treat."

This leaves open such basic questions as what we mean by "biological," not to mention "treat" or "really." A psychotherapist, presented with increasingly impressive biological research data on schizophrenia, shrugged his shoulders with "we'll ultimately be able to cure the sickest schizophrenics with the more refined psychotherapeutic techniques which we are beginning to understand," citing cases such as Atypical Manic and *I Never Promised You a Rose Garden* (Green, 1964). To each protagonist, thinking at the other level is like a medieval stopgap, to be employed only until the "real" cause and treatment are found. *But which level is "real"?* This question takes us right back to complex multilevel causality.

Each of the protagonists above commits a logical fallacy, or *system idolatry*, which is a practical version of the category error of confusing the part with the whole. Idolatry refers to worshiping a man-made creation instead of the greater reality or God that it represents— adherence to particular religious doctrine as the only "true way" being the classic example. This is the acceptance and nonacceptance principles (see Chapter 3) in both their healthy and unhealthy aspects: healthy in the need to define one's identity and what one stands for; unhealthy to the extent that it fosters closed-mindedness about alternative views.

Such system idolatry is equally prevalent even within the same broad level, like the psychological. Long-term psychotherapists presented with enduring change from a brief strategic intervention will often claim that the change is not "real"—presumably it did not cost a lot of money and take a lot of time, and did not utilize the same dynamics that long-term psychotherapies maintain are essential. Similar examples are legion and they pervade the entire human condition.

The most obvious logical fallacy is selective attention/inattention. The biologist conveniently ignored such cases as Atypical Manic and Grandma Is Depressed, which could have made him a "believer" of something quite different. The psychotherapist similarly ignored cases like Myxedema Madness, and the many schizophrenics who do as well on haloperidol as the former had done on thyroid replacement. What is most intriguing is how intensely the polar opposites are held against one another, even publicly, as in the 1984 APA debate about whether biological research has rendered psychodynamics obsolete! There are so many patients whose faulty "dynamics" disappear when the right medication is found, as well as biological treatment failures who improve when they are simply talked to, that it seems logically untenable to think in dichotomous terms. Yet, the either-or's continue, as exemplified by the nearly tragic case of Back Pain.

CASE 4. BACK PAIN: A SIMPLE VICIOUS CIRCLE

I was called to a medical ward for consultation with a Mrs. J, a chronic pain patient for whom no underlying medical cause could be identified. As I entered the ward I heard a piercing scream, followed by sounds of a scuffle occurring at the far end of the hall. Several ward attendants were dragging a young lady by her legs out of a tenth-floor window from which she had attempted to jump. This was Mrs. J. She had just been informed for the first time that a psychiatrist was being brought in on her case. Terminating a vicious tirade with statements that she would under no conditions talk with a "shrink," she was involuntarily detained to a high-security mental health unit since protection must always remain the number one priority. After she calmed down she was willing to talk, but adamantly maintained her denial of anything resembling emotional problems. All she could talk about was the severity of chronic low back pain which had resisted all attempts at diagnosis and therapeutic relief, and her bitter resentment of medical personnel who told her it was all in her head.

Among other things, this patient was a victim of the professional version of what I call the *either-or syndrome* — *either* there is a clearly defined or definable physical cause that can then be treated by a physical means, *or* it must be psychological, in which case only psychotherapy can be expected to help. This assumption is logical only following traditional mechanistic causality, and cases such as this illustrate the absurdity of this old model. As complex biopsychosocial causality gradually replaces mechanism, I hope and expect that a psychiatrist will be consulted from the very beginning in a complex case like this, with the result that different specialists then cooperate from the beginning in search of the approaches most likely to provide relief.

Indeed, no biological cause had been identified, and the workup had been exhaustive and more than adequate. This does not mean that there was no physical cause, only none *that could be identified and treated with current techniques*. It is well known that even mild stress on muscle and tendon attachments can be excruciatingly painful, and that these will not show up on X ray. Intense pain, exaggerated by emotional discounting, leads to anxiety, anxiety leads to guarding, guarding puts stress on any presumed locus of pain that in principle might be there, creating worse pain, which creates worse anxiety, etc. This classic simple causal loop, nearly identical to that discussed in Chapter 1, is illustrated in Figure 2.1.

In a causal loop, whichever cause is more basic or "real" is not only impossible to determine, but often meaningless. *Treatment can occur at*

Figure 2.1. Back pain: A vicious-circle model

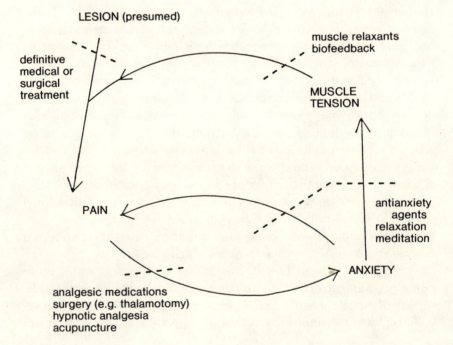

LESION (presumed)

muscle relaxants
biofeedback

definitive
medical or
surgical
treatment

MUSCLE
TENSION

PAIN

antianxiety
agents
relaxation
meditation

analgesic medications
surgery (e.g. thalamotomy)
hypnotic analgesia
acupuncture

ANXIETY

either level, equally definitively. The removal of a physical lesion will of course relieve the source of the anxiety, thereby breaking the circle, but no such lesion was identifiable in this particular case. However, if the anxiety and guarding are resolved by appropriate relaxation, meditation, biofeedback, or hypnotic techniques, the natural healing process is allowed to occur on its own.

Simple explanation with some reassurance and relaxation approaches were readily acceptable to this patient, with relief progressing to an end point of only mild chronic discomfort within a several-week period. Psychosocial conflicts were obvious to the examiner, as they had been to the referring physicians, but the patient was not receptive to any further intervention. The result was considered satisfactory.

EMOTIONAL OVERREACTIVITY AND "HYPOGLYCEMIA": A COMPLEX VICIOUS-CIRCLE MODEL FOR A COMPLEX DISORDER

The concept of hypoglycemia is widely used and often abused, and straddles the zones of life-threatening medical illness and psychosocial fad. I offer it as an example *par excellence* of the biopsychosocial model, showing reciprocal circular interactions between many biological, psychological, and social factors that cannot be reduced to only one single cause. Yet, the various factors remain specific enough to permit their being diagrammed (Fig. 2.2).

Hypoglycemia as a "cause" of or important contributing factor to neurotic and character disorders was first proposed by Harris (1936), whose paper remains a classic. Numerous references up to now have confirmed the prevalence of severe diet abuse in patients with impaired affect containment, and many cases cited where simply correcting the abusive eating pattern has led to therapeutic change as impressive as Beulah's thyroid replacement and discontinuing caffeine in the first case of this chapter. Whatever the primary cause, there is a relatively characteristic symptom picture as described below.

Symptomatology, while varied, most commonly consists of a mild, often subclinical, chronic depression characterized by fatigue and impaired motivation that is then punctuated by acute episodes of extreme dysphoria (blind rage, panic, suicidal despair, or equivalent) that occurs in response to objectively minor psychiatric stresses. There is an

Figure 2.2. Emotional hyperreactivity: A complex vicious-circle model

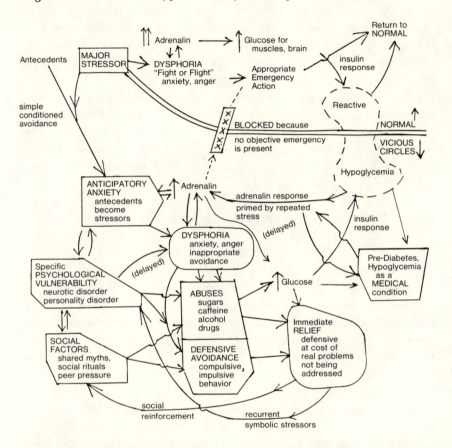

overall decrement in the patient's ability to cope with stress. Charac-teristically, these patients eat irregularly, abuse alcohol, and consume large amounts of caffeine.

In my experience, common psychiatric diagnoses are dysthymic disorder (though the depression is atypical); personality disorders with passive-aggressive, borderline, histrionic, and avoidant features; the varieties of alcoholism; and varieties of antisocial and explosive per-sonality. All are characterized by impulsive behavior in response to intolerable feelings, which the patient later regrets. Fredericks (1976) is the most recent proponent of wide use of the hypoglycemia concept, supported by the palliative relief that so many such patients find in hypoglycemic dieting even when there is a minimally disturbed glucose tolerance test.

The question often raised is to what extent hypoglycemia is causally related to these mental disorders. The classic abnormal test is illustrated in Figure 2.3, with a sharp but transient drop in blood sugar occurring between the second and fourth hours pc. Supporting the idea of hypoglycemia as causally related to mental disorders are the following correlates:

1) such patients often have a family history of diabetes to a far greater extent than the average patient;
2) the severity of emotional symptoms seems to correlate with a) the *severity* of the drop — more severe when sugars reach the low forties or below; and/or b) the *rapidity* of the drop — the symptoms being worse if the hypoglycemia occurs one hour rather than four hours pc; and
3) these patients often find profound, even dramatic relief from their emotional lability when they follow a strict hypoglycemic diet designed to moderate blood sugar fluctuations toward a more stable level.

Arguing against the causal relevance of the hypoglycemic concept are equally impressive data:

1) during the height of the emotional crisis, even when clearly related to diet abuse, immediate blood sugar determination is usually within the normal range;
2) the true hypoglycemia, when it occurs, is only transient, rarely lasting longer than an hour, whereas the emotional stress is often quite prolonged;
3) the degree of hypoglycemia is not often sufficient to cause *true* hypoglycemic symptoms, those of adrenergic hyperactivity, confusion, tremor, convulsions, or coma;
4) some patients experience the classic symptoms described with normal glucose tolerance tests, yet still demonstrate a dramatic response to hypoglycemic diet sometimes approaching cure;

Figure 2.3. The glucose tolerance curve

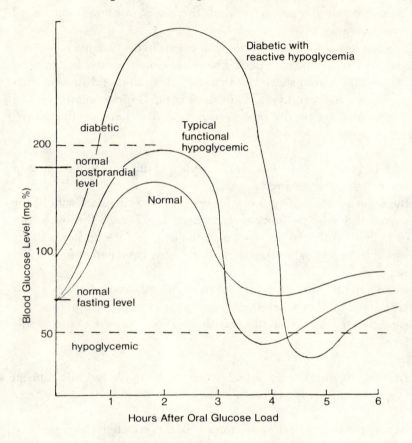

5) often victims of this disorder, while overreacting to minor stress, may cope adequately with a *major* stress involving major threat to self or family. I would not expect this to occur if the blood sugar at such times was seriously impaired.

Clearly there must be many other factors at work, and the word *hypoglycemia* may be inappropriate. Standard medical criteria for the diagnosis require a glucose level below 50 mg % accompanied by adrenergic symptoms. Hofeldt, Adler, and Herman (1975) comment that many normal individuals will approach these criteria and still not suffer any meaningful psychiatric symptoms. Yager and Young (1974) further discuss the faddish implications of the concept, arguing against its having any meaningful medical validity.

The syndrome might better be labeled *dysadrenalism*. The episodic dysphoria is compatible with discharge of epinephrine, which leads to an inappropriate fight or flight reaction; e.g., a patient responds to a snide remark or a dirty look from his wife as if a man-eating tiger were after him. The chronic depression so common between such episodes could be seen as a depletion state. An oversimplified yet still highly complex vicious-circle model is proposed, and illustrated in Figure 2.2.

Above the double line in this diagram is depicted the normal psychophysiological response to a major life-threatening trauma. There is an immediate intense dysphoric reaction resembling intense fear and/or anger, which ideally leads to appropriate emergency fight or flight reactions and resolution of the threat. Accompanying the dysphoric reaction in a closed causal loop is an outpouring of epinephrine (adrenalin), which both follows from and fuels the emotional reaction. A direct effect of the adrenalin is to stimulate glucose secretion, which provides more emergency food for muscles and brain. By normal negative feedback, once the threat is over, an insulin response will drop glucose levels to normal, and quite likely lead to a transient reactive hypoglycemia.

By simple conditioned avoidance, experience of multiple major stressors will lead to anticipatory anxiety that can accompany any chance antecedent of the major stressor. Thus, antecedents become stressors and are experienced as if they were cause of a major emergency even when there is none. Because no objective emergency exists, appropriate emergency reaction is meaningless and decisive problem solving is irrelevant by the very definition of the situation. Few have suffered so many stressors of such magnitude to cause this tragic effect, but victims of prolonged child abuse as well as wartime post-traumatic stress disorders can certainly illustrate this dynamic.

Now consider the role of diet abuse. Ingestion of either sucrose, glucose, caffeine, or alcohol have in common an immediate rise in postprandial blood sugar to higher than normal levels, which by normal negative feedback leads to an insulin response and a postprandial hypoglycemic episode, in a curve similar to that in Figure 2.3.

By similar normal negative feedback, the adrenals are stimulated by the hypoglycemia to secrete adrenalin, which in a severe episode causes the classic dysphoric symptoms of anxiety, tremor, and sweating. Thus, even in a healthy individual, diet abuse has the potential to increase vulnerability to fight or flight reactions in the absence of objective danger, since the adrenals are more "primed" to secrete adrenalin.

True hypoglycemia, often a prediabetic condition, simply exaggerates this response. Immediate rise in sugar is often much higher, even to the point of "sweet urine," and the resulting drop is to levels associated with transient mental confusion, followed by the catastrophic adrenalin response. *Rather than being a single or root cause, then, real hypoglycemia is simply a condition that exaggerates complex circular interactions to which we are all potentially vulnerable.*

An especially vicious circle is illustrated in the center part of the diagram. The immediate relief obtained through the abuses — a direct pharmacological effect of alcohol, the psychological "breast substitute," and the immediate resolution of hypoglycemia provided by glucose — parallels the infant who has just been nursed. This is a powerful positive reinforcer that increases the tendency to such abuse any time the dysphoria recurs. The dysphoria, equally "true" as a causal outcome of the abuse, is delayed sufficiently so the effects of classically conditioned avoidance are trivial compared to the reinforcement provided by the more immediate relief. There is a clear potential for escalation and deterioration that characterizes most addictive disorders.

Now consider the role of specific psychological vulnerabilities, those that are classically associated with neurotic and personality disorders. A common feature is inability to handle certain types of stress, with only symbolic stressors leading to inappropriate fight or flight reactions similar if not identical to the hyperadrenalism just described. According to psychodynamic theories, classic defensive avoidance mechanisms are employed, often at an unconscious level, with compulsive and impulsive behaviors resulting. These follow a classic pattern of tension, compulsive behavior leading to relief, and recurrent tension. Even without disordered sugar metabolism, there is a similar vicious circle in which the immediate defensive relief powerfully reinforces the avoidance mechanism, while the even more tragic result catches up with the patient only later — perpetuation of the disorder by virtue of the real problems having not been addressed. In actual clinical practice, *diet abuse and defensive avoidance go hand in hand to such a degree that they can rarely be separated, and the two complex circles merge.*

Adding to the complexity of the system are social factors: Many alcoholic patients lament that attempts at sobriety may require an entire change in social context, as their drinking buddies will often not make the same change at the same time. Often they are ill-prepared for such a massive upheaval. It has long been recognized that potent intervention against alcohol dependence can sometimes be accomplished only in cooperation with the patient's social network.

According to this model, it is meaningless to talk about any one input as the true or "real" cause. Research studies by Anthony et al. (1973) demonstrated that "reactive hypoglycemia is almost invariably accompanied by significant personality disorder" (p. 674), specifying parameters of this disorder along lines similar to those discussed above. They summarize the diffusion of causality as follows: "It may also be argued that a common preexisting personality pattern predisposes the patients to the development of hypoglycemia . . . hypoglycemia may then produce the exacerbation of this preexisting personality pattern to a pathological level. A definitive statement of the direction of causality between hypoglycemia and personality disorders cannot be made on the basis of data presented in this study alone" (p. 674).

The beauty of the model presented in Figure 2.2 is that we do not need to become embroiled in either-or conflicts, being either for or against a concept such as hypoglycemia. Our attention is drawn to a *search for focal points.* These can be found at many levels: Where true hypoglycemia is present, eating in such a way as to minimize the fluctuations in sugar level (i.e., with a hypoglycemic diet) attenuates the adrenalin response and modulates the inappropriate dysphoric response to stress. The result is the improved frustration tolerance that is so often found with patients on hypoglycemic diets. To a lesser degree, the same response should be found in any human being. Similarly, if specific psychological vulnerabilities are protected, covered over, or resolved, improved frustration tolerance will similarly result. There will be less impulse toward abusive avoidance techniques and more joy in simple living.

Anticipatory anxiety may be dealt with in some individuals by simple behavioral techniques such as desensitization. In others, it requires modification of social habits that contribute to the vicious circle, or prolonged exploratory psychotherapy and working through. For still others, the simple discipline provided by new eating habits has psychological implications, providing structure in other far-reaching areas of their lives. Which will prove to be the best focal point for a given patient will vary. The point is that if complex biopsychosocial interaction makes the search for primary causes hopeless, we are rewarded with a corresponding flexibility in potential points of intervention. This is the essence of the biopsychosocial model and the essential point of this volume.

While it will rarely influence the choice of treatment, I do order a formal glucose tolerance test in the following situations:

1) when I suspect hypoglycemia of sufficient significance that the patient will be impressed, motivating him to take better care of himself;
2) any stigmata of borderline diabetes mellitus or strong family history of this (and similarly but to a lesser degree with obesity and alcoholism);
3) *patient's request* — many patients have been denied glucose tolerance tests by physicians because "there is no evidence for it."

I know of at least three who subsequently demonstrated blood sugar levels in the 30s. With defensive medicine so prevalent, we may pay a high price for such rigid mechanistic thinking.

TREATMENT GUIDELINES

It is not my purpose here to give specific guidelines for appropriate application of psychobiology, such as use of antidepressants, antipsychotics, or lithium; nor to offer such guidelines regarding treatment using specific psychosocial modalities. These are competently presented in all modern psychiatric texts. An especially useful approach to all three levels is presented by Lewis and Usdin (1982) and choice of therapeutic modality and theoretical system will be the topic of Chapter 8.

Whatever the treatment, appropriate planning will take into consideration certain coherent issues. First is a benefit/detriment analysis. In addition to the potential benefits we must ask whether these benefits are short-term or long-term, and what the costs will be in achieving them. As far as risks are concerned, and as exemplified by the use of psychotropic medications, we need to ask several questions:

1) What are the immediate side effects (dry mouth with antidepressants, tremor and sedation with antipsychotics)?
2) What are the long-term problems (tardive dyskinesia with antipsychotics, kidney disorders with lithium)?
3) Could the treatment prevent resolution of the problem by sidestepping another issue that is potentially treatable, as exemplified by Coffee Addict?
4) Is there potential for addiction, not only biological but *psychological* addiction such as the case of the Perfect Primal (p. 45)?
5) Are risks imposed by *idiosyncratic connotations*?

For example, for one patient, prescribing an antidepressant symbolizes comfort from a benign authority, but for another it implies that his feelings are wrong, bad, or defective, leading to increased defensive avoidance and worsening of his symptoms. Long-term problems are not only biological, but include regressive dependency and social and financial costs in the case of long-term psychotherapy.

In general, I consider biological intervention indicated in the following cases:

1) when the problem appears to be a true physical disorder or illness unrelated to psychological conflicts, as evidenced by its symptoms, course, and family history;
2) even if it is psychological in dominant cause, if (a) the symptoms are so severe that they override psychological interventions, in which case the biological treatment may enable the patient to work, (b) it is simply the easiest way to go (benefit/detriment analysis);
3) when rapid control is necessary (i.e., when the first priority is protection).

Despite biopsychosocial unity, the biological approach is probably appropriate for pervasive disorders affecting the entire system.

Psychological disorders, by contrast, more often manifest as conflict between two parts of a person that cannot be separated in space, time, or even in principle. Any medication acting on one part would also act on the other. No matter how specific the pathway a particular drug may act upon, if both parts of an intrapsychic conflict use the same pathways, this problem remains; both end up taking the drug when only one is felt to need it! (This will be discussed more fully in Chapters 3 through 5.)

Psychological structure is an abstraction that can never be measured or tested, but remains useful for understanding personality disorders. It is given research support by data that show certain aspects of the central nervous system to mature at particular critical periods of development, requiring certain types of sensory nutriment at those times. Absence of appropriate parenting, major trauma, or even medical disorder at those critical periods could lead to a failure in development well described by the psychodynamic term *defect*. No clear definitive biological treatment would seem appropriate for this, unless we are able to develop a way to temporarily restore the lost plasticity of the original critical period. In this case a combination of biological and hypnotic technique might repair the original defect. Long-term psychotherapy may partially achieve this end.

Biopsychosocial dilemmas are discussed further in Chapter 6, with the social dimension being clarified further in Chapter 4.

3

The Psychological
Level: Basic Humanness

OVERVIEW

This chapter addresses the psychological level, the inner subjective awareness where all of us live our private lives, along with its external correlate, interpersonal behavior. It elaborates the relevance and clinical utilization of the many untestable intangibles that contribute to this level: free choice, motivation, acceptance/nonacceptance dilemmas, and the even more subtle components of human value priorities and the vicissitudes of human language. It is difficult to think of these in the same terms as matter-energy, extended in space and time. They appear instead to follow their own rules. The purpose of this chapter is to abstract the key features of this level, and illustrate them with clinical case material and discussion to assist the clinician in its utilization and clarify its place in the broader realm of biopsychosocial psychiatry.

The primary characteristic of the psychological level is *free choice*, a little-understood agency that is capable of breaking most of the rules of scientific psychiatry. Whether free will arises from yet unknown laws that govern all natural substance (Beahrs, 1977a; Freud, 1916/1979; Spinoza, 1677/1951) or whether mind is an "independent entity" that transcends but regulates matter-energy (LeShan & Margenau, 1982, p. 242) does not need to concern the practicing clinician. In either case, we must work with free choice as a basic given. The free choice of another person demands our inviolable respect, even while we make all reasonable effort to limit its effects when destructive and influence its direction toward more desirable outcomes.

This and the following two chapters elaborate on the special features of the psychological level. This chapter clarifies the importance of acceptance/nonacceptance dilemmas and a patient's overall frame of reference. Chapter 4 more explicitly addresses the dilemmas of interpersonal control, with the need to respect a patient's autonomy while doing all we can to effectively influence him toward change. In Chapter 5 we find that all of the qualities we attribute to consciousness — free will, motivation, values, etc. — are not unified, but exist at different levels simultaneously within the same individual. Only at this point will several key elements of the psychological level become more clear, most specifically the difference between voluntary and involuntary choice, psychodynamic mechanisms, and intrapsychic conflict.

The most important contributing factor to free choice is motivation. Motivation provides the energetics for higher human activity. If man is likened to a complex machine, motivation is the "psychic energy" that drives it. Both psychoanalytic conflict theory and behavior therapy grant appropriately high priority to drives and motivation and have made commendable strides toward putting these on firm scientific ground. But they have proven inept at dealing with certain slippery intangibles that have equal or greater importance in determining the course of human living.

These intangibles include human value priorities, cherished irrational and personal styles, idiosyncratic personality quirks, pride, and the many ways a person tries to save face. Even if these were held constant, a different person might put an opposite connotation onto the same word, phrase, or concept, and the resulting change in motivation might lead to an outcome far different from expected. There is no way that these untestable intangibles can be measured or tested *in toto*; therefore, they defy scientific specification. Yet these subtle motivational issues are what raise humankind above the rest of the animal kingdom, reflecting as they do the intricacies of language. The untestable intangibles in human motivation constitute the third fundamental root of uncertainty in mental health. Forever beyond science, they are often the most important determinants of human behavior, and essential elements in whether and how psychiatric intervention can be helpful.

Within the realm of human motivation are three distinguishable dichotomies. Closest to science is the *pleasure principle* of Freud (1916/1979) stated more clearly by Spinoza (1677/1951): We seek pleasure and avoid pain. Extending this to a higher level of abstraction leads to the good/evil dichotomy. While we usually seek good and avoid evil, we do not say that pleasure is always good or pain always bad. In fact, ethics probably arose from the awareness of the two levels of motivation and the need to differentiate between them (Beahrs, 1977a). Already far beyond science, all of history illustrates the importance of good and evil to mental health. Just as relevant to our study is a third dichotomy at yet a higher level of abstraction, often referred to by the slippery term *OKness*. Pleasure or pain, good or evil — any can be OK or not OK in a person's overall outlook, the importance of which was recognized and best described by Berne (1972) in his concept of existential position. Meaning "acceptance" or "endorsement," the word *OK* is used in two senses: to denote a broad state of being that dominates most of a person's behavior and to qualify whether we should endorse or repudiate a more specific action or moral position. In my practice, the acceptance/nonacceptance dilemmas pervade most of the psychological level.

A working "acceptance principle" often proves to have considerable clinical utility as well as a central role in personal well-being. Acceptance does not mean endorsing specific activity that we call evil, that which we should continue to abhor and do our best to modify. It does, however, mean that we endorse the nature of basic humanness with all of its foibles, recognizing that it contains much potential for what we call sin. It also implies living with what is, as opposed to what should be. In lay terms, it is often called a philosophical attitude. It is close to what I earlier termed a *state of faith*, a precondition for healthy living whose antonym is depression in its many forms and transformations (Beahrs, 1977a; Lowen, 1972; Roberts, 1974). Equally important to mental health is an antithetical principle of nonacceptance, existing alongside its converse in a creative tension that no scientific principles can resolve. Acceptance is most clearly appropriate to what cannot be changed but simply is; whatever constitutes our basic being, that of others, and all of "what is" that we take as a given.

Ideally, nonacceptance applies to what is not given, but to what can and should be changed. Specific destructive actions are the clearest case in point. Since the two domains are most difficult to tease apart from one another, it is inevitable that they will be confused.

Must psychopathology arises from covert rejection of important aspects of basic being. When we try to "get rid of" inviolable aspects of our basic being, they return as symptoms that torment us and can poison our lives at many levels. Often the same patients will experience destructive voluntary behaviors as if they were a basic given, feeling that their symptom relieves them of responsibility. Reframing is the primary therapeutic vehicle for promoting acceptance, while confrontation is its equivalent where negative judgment and behavior control are needed. Interpretation, clarification, and information all heighten the patient's awareness, fostering a healthy sense of being in charge.

The importance of reframing is illustrated by the first case of this chapter, Luxury Cruise, and appears again and again throughout this volume. The second case, Perfect Primal, illustrates the disastrous effect that even subtle nonacceptance can have when inappropriately applied to an important aspect of one's basic being. Affect-containment strategies, such as the body continuum and cognitive therapy, are offered as a corrective. Case 3, War Veteran, exemplifies the all-too-frequent confusion of categories that we so often see in personality disorders. Here, confrontation and control of negative behavior proved equally essential to fostering a healthy acceptance.

Many issues are raised by the fuzziness of the acceptance/nonacceptance dilemmas, their dominating role in determining the quality of life, and the awesome power that a skilled psychiatric therapist can wield in this area by such simple devices as reframing. First is the problem of evil, especially as we see it in the consulting room in the form of self-destructive aspects of personality or moral lacunae harmful not only to the patient but to loved ones and society at large. This topic will be dealt with throughout this volume along with issues of social control, vengeance, and the need for forgiveness.

Tension between psychological and objective realities also presents troublesome choice dilemmas, even in the rare case where the two can adequately be distinguished. Many argue that accepting the cold facts or true horror of "reality" is a precondition to any further therapeutic growth (Goulding & Goulding, 1979; Lowen, 1983). Freud (1916/1979), however, argued that "psychological reality" sometimes differed from what actually happened, and could be treated as if it were objective. Erickson (Beahrs, 1971) hypnotically "added" new constructs to past history as needed so that the negative psychological past could be changed to a better one. Roberts (1974) even claims that we "create our own reality," carrying the obligation to make our reality into one that feels good and works. As with most such arguments it is probably either-and; the question to be addressed is when and in what situation to use which approach.

Common to all of these acceptance/nonacceptance dilemmas is an overriding need to find some protective structure, both individual and social, to define who we are, where we are going, what kind of behaviors are acceptable and what are not, and what we are to believe and not to believe. With absolute "truth" devastated by the many roots of uncertainty and increasingly replaced by utility, the need for a way to organize our belief structure in a manner that is both scientifically acceptable, useful, and maximally protective becomes more critical than ever. With increasing contempt for old value systems and dogmatic morality, along with recognition of the power of reframing, there is a similar need to put ethics on firm, solid, and protective ground, yet on a foundation flexible enough to meet the new demands.

This structure can be found at a new level — the presumption. *Presumption* is defined exactly as in legal theory, like the presumption of "innocent until proven guilty." The moral presumption (Brill, 1979) states that chosen agreed-upon value priorities or moral edicts can be held valid unless "proven" otherwise. One can accept a particular code of ethics like the Ten Commandments, recognizing that occasionally one tenet may infringe upon another, in which case a difficult moral choice must be made. The moral presumption simply puts the burden of proof on he who would violate a tenet. For example, war is evil but Naziism demonstrates that by *not* violating that tenet in rare cases a worse evil could follow. With that presumption, fewer wars would be fought, but those that are would be on more solid moral ground.

The following case presentation illustrates the powers of the acceptance/nonacceptance dilemmas, and how simply helping a patient to change the meaning he attributes to a specific situation may lead to positive change that can pervade his entire life. This is what Watzlawick, Weakland, and Fisch (1974) called the "gentle art of reframing" (p. 100), the type of focal point most frequently successful when working with a patient at the psychological level.

CASE 1. LUXURY CRUISE

Ivan was a 34-year-old white male engineer in ongoing exploratory psychotherapy to relieve troubling personal inhibitions. He came to the current psychotherapy session acutely anxious, in dread of an impending Christmas visit to his mother 2,000 miles away.

> A classic "Jewish mother." She means well but just has to do everything she can for me, even though I am more competent than she. She gives me $20 to go out on the town every night, even though I make three times as much as she does. She even salts my food, although I don't particularly like salt. And the more I protest to her that I am not only a grown man but an extremely competent one at that, the more she tries to pamper and baby me. It is oppressive, insufferable, and intolerable, and I am just simply helpless to do anything about it.

This is similar in several ways to the case of Problematic Punctuation in Chapter 1, illustrating circular causality. First, the person seeking help is actually seeking help to change the behavior of another individual, this time one living across the country and thereby not able to see the same therapist even if she wanted to. Second, all techniques already employed by the patient have either failed or actually made matters worse. Toward relieving a self-perpetuating vicious circle, a strategic therapeutic double bind was prescribed for this patient.

Ivan was encouraged to go ahead with his plans to visit his mother, but to carry out his vacation with a very specific attitude. He was to imagine that he was on a luxury cruise and that his mother's entire reason for existing was to wait on him hand and foot to ensure that he had the most exquisitely luxurious experience possible for any creature on earth to enjoy. Whatever his mother offered, the patient was to thank her profusely and commend himself on how fortunate he was to have such a fine mother.

However, Ivan was never to be fully satisfied; he was always to ask for more. If his mother sprinkled a little salt on part of his hot dish he was to ask for pepper on another, and perhaps a dash of oregano or thyme on his salad or garlic bread. If a rare seafood dish was served he was to ask for some caviar. If he was given $20 to go out on the town, he was to thank her profusely but to ask, "Are you aware that prices have gone up? Would it be too much to ask if you could spare

$30?" A gleam in Ivan's eye suggested that I had probably hit an effective focal point. "I think I can really get into this game."

Preparatory discussion suggested either of two probable reactions on his mother's part. On the one hand, she might continue to indulge her son and even escalate the behavior. In this case he was simply to relax and enjoy it, to savor the delights of high living as if he were on a luxury cruise, and to return home relaxed and refreshed.

Just as likely, however, Ivan's mother might become impatient with his indulgences. She might become fed up with his insatiable demands and say, "Don't you think it's about time you grew up? You've been dependent on me all these years, despite my having given you the best education that money can buy. As much as I care about you, I just have to draw the line sometime. A person has to be weaned."

Should the latter come about, the patient is to avoid at all costs any angry exclamation such as, "That's what I have been trying to get you to do for years!!" Instead he is to contritely acknowledge the correctness of her views; that, in fact, he does enjoy being taken care of, and given "such a perfect mother" it is hard to do anything other than relax and enjoy it. While the real world is quite cold and cruel, he nonetheless "realizes" painfully that her statement is what he in fact needs to do, and that he will "try."

This is the classic *therapeutic double bind* described by Haley (1963) and his strategic followers. A frustrating negative situation in which nothing seems right simply is reframed so that nothing can be wrong —without any change in the actual facts of the situation.

What really happened? Ivan returned from vacation saying that he had not employed the luxury cruise game because he felt no need to. He had felt remarkably comfortable with his mother and engaged in very few of his former push-pull games, instead enjoying an adult heart-to-heart talk with her for the first time in his life that both found gratifying.

REFRAMING: THE FOUNDATION
OF PSYCHOTHERAPY

The benefits of Ivan's "luxury cruise" can be understood from several perspectives. Since he actually employed no specific strategies once his trip was underway, the positive outcome is best understood in terms of a change in attitude, a shift from nonacceptance to acceptance. This is positive reframing. Instead of dreading the encounter with his mother, instead of being prepared to struggle and plead with her from the point of view of a petulant child, he was looking forward to having a good time. Hence, he probably came across more as the mature adult that he in fact was, and from that point of view more likely perceived his mother similarly. The gratifying rapprochement that followed became virtually inevitable.

The power of reframing lies in the attitude/behavior transformation from avoidance to acceptance or even approach. As illustrated by the luxury cruise that Ivan never took, this can be accomplished simply by giving a different meaning to a reality that remains the same. What has changed is only the motivational structure, that which is sought or avoided. But this can alter dramatically the entire dynamic structure of the individual. Something that the patient formerly was terrified of he now feels comfortable with or even likes; thus, he will no longer need to employ the same defense against what was dreaded. With its motivational underpinnings removed, a symptom simply may disappear.

The profound paradoxical element in Ivan's "luxury cruise" is best understood by speculating on what would have happened if the patient had actually employed the therapeutic double bind. The most desired outcome would have been for his mother to confront his dependency and assert his need to take care of himself and assume more responsibility, in which case he would have agreed apologetically but would have told her it would be "most difficult." In other words, we know that the more the patient pleaded for autonomy, the more his mother would have smothered him. And if he overtly had sponged on her, the more she would have been inclined to wean him from his prolonged childish dependency.

This paradox reflects neither perversity nor oppositional behavior, but the massive ambivalence normally felt by both parties when a dependent offspring leaves home. On the one hand, the adult desires to be a man with all of the burdens as well as the joys of his autonomy; on the other hand, the child in him wants to be taken care of forever. Mother is equally ambivalent. She wants him to remain her little child forever, but she equally wants him to mature and make his mark in the world despite the pain of separation that this must entail. It is neither hypocrisy nor gamesmanship, but the simple fact that a healthy person may want one thing *and* its opposite, honestly and with equal intensity.

To argue the advantage of either side may threaten the other, which is then likely to come forth in response as a corrective. Paradox is not just reverse psychology; it is better considered as "straight talk" to a part of the patient's self that is in the background, and that so far has not been given adequate voice or taken seriously. This understanding anticipates the different levels of consciousness or ego states, the topic of Chapter 5 (see also Beahrs, 1982b).

Not only is reframing effective and efficient, the associated paradoxical twists are often fun for patient and therapist alike. By respecting another's basic being, which can rarely be changed to any great degree, it is also the least invasive and most respectful of other people's autonomy. For these reasons, reframing should be considered as the cornerstone of all psychotherapy.

Almost all psychotherapeutic techniques utilize some reframing when they are effective, not only the strategic and paradoxical approaches. Dollard and Miller (1950) pointed out the profound element of reframing in a psychoanalyst's initial response to a patient's imagined "worst catastrophe." If the analyst can be so calm, this implies that the problem cannot be so horrible. Elements of reframing also pervade the very core of awareness and affect-containment strategies, which will be discussed in more depth. To assist the therapist in this "gentle art," Table 3.1 presents a reframing list, a brief and partial compilation of concepts with negative connotations along with how they are often reframed, thereby giving therapy new direction.

CASE 2. PERFECT PRIMAL

Donna, a middle-aged white female professional, sought counseling for symptoms of burnout — chronic anxiety and fatigue, resentment of her professional duties, occasional crying spells, and increasing impairment of both her professional and personal relationships. As there had been minor depression of over two year's duration, the diagnosis was dysthymic disorder (neurotic depression). Her activist nonpsychiatric therapist considered her difficulties due to fear of in-

TABLE 3.1
Partial Reframing List

Concept to be Reframed		Often Reframed as
AFFECTIVE STATES	Dysphoria	Emotional nutriment; Signal; Affect bridge to the "unconscious"
	Fear	Excitement; Protector; Signal of danger
	Anger	Protector, defense; power, enforcer; Signal
	Depression	Rest, recuperation, other feeling
	Pain	Excitement; Signal; Temperature, other sensation
SITUATIONS	Setback; Risk, danger	Opportunity, Challenge
	Symptom, affliction	Protector; Special advantage
	Psychological defect	Delayed maturation, misused skill
	Symbiosis	Loving; Sharing
BEHAVIORS	Resistance, distancing	Autonomy
	Mistrust, paranoia	Caution, watchfulness, protectiveness,
	Controlling	Safe, Cautious; Moral, ethical
	Crazy, psychotic	Creative, Imaginative; occasionally, bad
	Manipulation	Skill; Leadership ability; Tact, diplomacy
	Disruption	Watchguard function, "Paul Revere"
	Gullible	Trusting, flexible
	Aggression	Defense
	(many abuses)	Fun-loving; Recreation
	Badness	Protective; other (sick, crazy, angry)
ATTRIBUTIONS	Rigidity; dogmatism	Integrity; Decisiveness, independence
	Wishy-washy	Flexible; Open-minded
	Dependence	Loving, caring, sharing

TABLE 3.1
(*continued*)

Concept to be Reframed		Often Reframed as
	Abnormal, freakish	Unique, innovative
	Guilt-ridden, compulsive	Moral, ethical; Conscientious
	Narcissistic, egotistic	Proud; Self-reliant; Independent
	Bland, boring	Stable, dependable
	Unstable	Interesting
	Annoying, irritating	Stimulating, exciting
	Inferior	Simply human
OTHER	Negative ego state	Original function, usually protective
	"Stuck"	Reviewing options; taking stock

NO REFRAMING FOR BLATANTLY DESTRUCTIVE & DISRESPECTFUL BEHAVIORS: These are simply UNACCEPTABLE

tense feelings, specifically anger and grief, that led to her keeping these bottled up within her where they festered and gnawed at all aspects of her life. The cure: to get them out.

Utilizing experiential techniques with masterful skill, the therapist encouraged the patient to ventilate, abreact, and "get it out" in many forms: She pounded pillows while angrily castigating real and imagined oppressors; she cried bitterly over emotional deprivations by loved ones decades ago. Each time she experienced profound relief and immediately afterwards returned to her former level of functioning. But the dysphoric feelings always returned—each time with a more demanding quality and an even greater sense of urgency.

After a year of such therapy the patient was feeling worse: chronic anxiety and disturbed sleep were increasing, and she became so impaired in her professional duties that she was forced to take an untimely sabbatical. Her personal relationships were disastrous. In short, she was functionally incapacitated. She continued aiming for bigger and better "primals," valued almost as if they were a form of art in themselves, yet all the while, her condition deteriorated.

FEELING-ORIENTED STRATEGIES

False causality in this case is exquisitely subtle. The therapist was entirely correct in his assumption that Donna was terrified of intense feelings, that her avoidance gave these feelings the power to dominate her life, and that what was needed was for her to learn to cope with them and utilize them more effectively. Here false causality is not at the level of structural fact, but of personal *attitude toward* this fact.

The implication of "getting it out" is that feelings are bad and should be gotten rid of, like excrement. An abreaction, often followed by relief, as in this case, may be sufficiently dramatic for the patient to desire further abreactions. But when the feelings recur, as they always will, the negative misattribution leads to their having an increased catastrophic quality, rendering them more dysphoric and pressing. The next primal is "bigger and better," and the relief even more dramatic, but the dysphoria is also more desperate when it comes back. An escalating vicious circle insidiously leads to progressive deterioration in the person's ability to contain affect and control behavior, even to the point that there is risk of major thought disorder. The regressive tendency can become sufficiently global to incapacitate the unfortunate individual.

Feeling-oriented work has been associated with depth therapy ever since the pioneering work of Breuer and Freud (1895/1955), and is often accompanied by intense subjective experience and vivid abreaction. For almost as long a time, conservative therapists have been wary of the risk for regressive dependency, illustrating this concern with cases such as the tragic Perfect Primal, and the recently more widespread phenomenon of cultism (see Chapter 6). Whether a feeling-oriented awareness strategy will be regressive or integrative boils down to the connotations derived from the feelings to be addressed. If they are negative, to be discharged or "gotten rid of," regression is the most likely outcome. If they are positive, to be experienced, integrated, contained, and directed; then growth and maturation will most likely follow.

An individual nearly identical to Perfect Primal was seen by a gestaltist, equally skilled at eliciting profound emotional experience and encouraging abreaction when necessary. That therapist, like that of Perfect Primal, asserted that the problem was how the patient handled feelings, but despite many superficial similarities in the resulting therapy the attitude he conveys is exactly the opposite of that of the first therapist. He sees feelings not as something to be "gotten rid of" at any level, but instead as basically positive, powerful, and constructive life forces that will naturally change to other feelings when simply permitted to be. They are to be *experienced fully*, contained, and integrated in a fully functioning individual. Instead of regressive deterioration of personality, this led to full maturation and growth.

Affect-Containment Strategies

A variety of experiential affect-containment strategies have been summarized in depth (Beahrs & Humiston, 1974). The fundamental rule is to fully experience by choice an uncomfortable dysphoric feeling. The feeling state is reframed as psychological nutriment and the patient is encouraged to "let happen whatever happens" — whether that means experiencing his dysphoria even more intensely or allowing it to change to something else — and to *do nothing*.

The subtle connotations of this directive are all positive. First, the feeling itself must be all right and possibly even the key to overcoming his disorder, or the (assumed) benevolent authority could not make such a recommendation. Second, to "let happen whatever happens" is a powerful endorsement of acceptance. Since the natural course of feelings is to flow from one another, change will inevitably occur when permitted. And third, by doing nothing, the patient makes the vital discovery that there is no necessary link between unpleasant feelings and destructive behavior — he permits the former and prevents the latter by choice.

When major mental illness is not present, this strategy will usually lead to spontaneous relief within 20 to 40 minutes, followed by evidence of hypnotic trance behavior. It is proposed as a formal "body awareness induction." In contrast to other hypnotic procedures, the therapy is in the induction itself rather than in the utilization of what follows. What is therapeutic is the corrective emotional experience itself — the patient's feeling the most feared emotion, and finding that he ends up feeling better, not worse. When trance utilization is still desired, the patient is highly receptive to an exploration of whatever underlies the original dysphoric mood. This follows from the very nature of the procedure.

A significant minority of patients will remain stuck, the dysphoric affect failing to resolve simply by letting it be fully experienced. One of two variants, then, can be employed: the two-chair techniques initially described by Perls (1969) or an *affect bridge* (Watkins, 1971), by which some original developmental trauma can be identified, abreacted, and worked through. The two-chair technique is intended to foster the simultaneous self-awareness of split-off and often warring psychological levels or ego states; integration can follow through internal diplomacy or a process of negotiation. In the affect bridge the dysphoria is the link between the here and now and the original situation. The affect bridge is a powerful antithesis to projective identification (see p. 79), disrupting the inappropriate link between old feelings and current relationships, returning instead to the source.

With a large case series I have found these strategies most potent in dysthymic disorder and other neurotic states, although high-level personality disorders may benefit equally from affect containment. Substance abuse, impulse control, and post-traumatic stress disorder also may benefit from body awareness experiential strategies, usually combined with their cognitive equivalents, as in Case 3 which follows.

Pure anxiety states, avoidant by very definition, are generally not positively affected by such an approach, though rarely are they worsened. Relaxation strategies like the relaxation response (Benson & Klipper, 1976) and biofeedback are more often helpful here, and interestingly, they are less effective with the depressive and dysphoric states just described. An important exception in clinical practice is when anxiety covers over an underlying mood disorder, where the body awareness approach will often still be the treatment of choice.

Only once have I found the containment-oriented awareness approach to have been clearly contraindicated in a nonpsychotic individual. In this case the affect bridge led to reactivating a deeply buried paranoid delusional system with boiling desires for vengeance against imaginary persecutors. A rapid and respectful switching of gears managed to avert further regression, and the patient was referred to a mental health center where responsibility could be diffused among many treatment personnel, and ego-building techniques used at many levels. While the risk may be rare statistically, cases like this and Perfect Primal remind us that potent techniques require not only skilled practitioners, but those with the protective background of professional training and certification.

LANGUAGE: THE POWER OF CONNOTATION

The tragic outcome of Perfect Primal can be attributed to the negative connotation of the uncomfortable feelings that were otherwise appropriately addressed as a focal point. This negative attribution, of course, fostered the patient's fear of the very feelings that she most needed to accept, leading to more avoidant behavior and a growing catastrophic attitude towards the feelings when they inevitably recurred. An escalating cycle of increased emotional pain and regressive dependency led to the tragic result. Although affect-containment approaches lead to superficially similar abreaction, they otherwise would have led to decrease in avoidance and increase in approach behavior and affect containment, resulting in integration, growth, and maturation. *The true focal point is the negative attribution that needs to be replaced by positive attribution of such an important aspect of one's basic being as his recurrent feeling states.*

Connotation often has capricious twists and turns, even in regard to specific words for which the meaning is not implied in dictionary definitions. The same is true with the implications of our actions. Prescribing a tricyclic antidepressant medication may imply a benevolent authority providing comfort to a patient and will facilitate the response. But to another it implies that our feelings are bad, something to be changed or gotten rid of—that can lead to a more subtle version of the same avoidance behavior that crippled Perfect Primal. Hence, psychological artifact may either help or hinder the treatment and it is hard to know in advance which direction the power of connotation will take.

For one patient, a biological explanation of his symptoms may provide a welcome face-saver but to another it may imply that he is defective and may promote shame, as well as his feeling that his very real emotional and moral struggles are being ignored. Similarly, a psychodynamic formulation will offer understanding and hope to one patient, rejuvenating his sense of power to constructive action, while to another it implies moral turpitude, responsibility, and guilt. The skillful psychotherapist will remain finely tuned to these nuances, so far from the purely scientific. Often, when other factors remain the same, these nuances will determine the very choice of treatment modality itself.

Healthy living appears to require a balance of many polar opposites in tension with one another at many levels, as illustrated in Figure 5.2 (p. 111). Each pole of a dichotomy has constructive (positive) and problematic (negative) aspects. For example, socioeconomic and political functioning require a balance of the conservative and liberal poles. Positive conservatism is simply an effort to protect and defend what is good in one's already existing life and social system. By contrast, negative conservatism is rigidly stifling to creativity and change, and in its extreme form becomes fascism or the internal tyranny of obsessive-compulsive disorder and other neurotic states. Positive liberalism is simply growth, maturation, and altruism, while negative liberalism is anarchy, destructiveness, and a unified standard of mediocrity. The French Revolution was a paradigm of negative liberalism, and the tragic paradox of much of today's liberal activism is implied in Haykin's (personal communication, 1981) barb, "Make peace or I'll kill you!"

Thus, acceptance in this case refers to the positive aspect of the pole in that the therapist's burden of responsibility is to help the patient shift the connotations, or implied meanings, so that his motivations will lead with less conflict in a more positive direction.

ACCEPTANCE/NONACCEPTANCE DILEMMAS

Acceptance and nonacceptance apply not only to specific connotations but also to the more pervasive states of being that Berne (1972) calls the *existential position*.

A person can experience unpleasant feelings that range from overwhelming grief to bitter despair and frustrated rage, all the time retaining his sense of the overall positivity of himself, others, and what is. In this sense, acceptance refers to the state of faith that provides meaning to life and fuel for constructive action in the face of adversity (Beahrs, 1977a; Roberts, 1974). Its antithesis can be depression (Lowen, 1972), despair (Kohut, 1971), or destructiveness (Fromm, 1973). These reflect nonacceptance as a state of being, exemplified in psychiatry by the affective, narcissistic, and paranoid disorders, respectively. When a person is in this kind of state everything is apt to feel ugly, and even normally pleasant feelings are tainted with a sense that things are simply not right. The source of existential nonacceptance often lies in the roots of vengeance and hanging on, the central dilemma of life discussed in the Epilogue. But a biological derangement may have a similar effect, as well as massive alterations in the social context.

Treatment can occur at equally as many levels, often different from that of dominant causality (see Chapter 2 for many examples). In any case, a psychiatrist is often called upon to help a patient relieve these states of nonacceptance. To do this, he may call upon a working principle increasingly dominant in the experiential, transactional, and hypnotic psychotherapies of the past two decades. I call this the *acceptance principle*: Everything that exists, including all human beings and all their aspects or parts, is to be accepted in its basic being, despite judgments about the ethics of certain behaviors.

To derive the acceptance principle, we begin to look at all that exists as polarity and paradox: For a proton there is an antiproton, for a male, a female, for the conscious, the unconscious, for good, evil. More importantly, even the same event, experience, or behavior can be considered in different ways that can lead to opposing positions or value judgments toward it and each can be "equally true" factually (see also Chapter 5).

This observation permits us to view any situation from perspectives that would emphasize either its positivity or negativity. We can dwell on the restrictiveness of our upbringing or the limits of our gender or innate abilities, and cry for "liberation," or we can choose to focus on the same as innate *assets* and develop these to the fullest. This viewpoint of the relationship of good and evil is the philosophical basis of reframing: a positive view is no more true than a negative one, but because it feels better and works better, it is preferred.

The greatest difficulty in implementing the acceptance principle arises from our appropriate fear of a "little Hitler" in ourselves and others — the potential for destructive aggression and denigration of the values that are so necessary for living cooperatively. G. Pascall (personal communication, 1979) raises this challenge most explicitly: "If you attempt to reconcile Adolph Hitler to the idea that any person or part of a person is OK, doesn't the very problem of evil evaporate?" The implication is that if we were to define an evildoer as basically OK we would then lose any rationale for fighting evil and it would fester and grow to levels first abhorrent and then intolerable, as during the 1930s.

We have trouble finding anything acceptable about that part of a person that sabotages all his attempts to better his life or to achieve healthier relationships and that reduces that person to a chronic mental patient or criminal. Yet, *looking for and finding* this acceptance in even the most negative aspects of life and validating it in a way that furthers more positive outcomes, is precisely what we must do if we are to be maximally effective.

Differentiating basic being from behaviors helps us to fulfill this task. It rarely runs counter to an offender's own assessment to confront the unacceptability of his negative behavior, and we can still support the individual's pride by respecting his basic being. Even where criminal justice is required for protection of society, it can be made clear that it is the *behavior* that is unacceptable, and decisive action is required to prevent its recurrence. While we are confronting and prohibiting a negative behavior, by respecting the original purpose of that behavior (usually protective), we can sometimes turn it into an asset (see also Chapter 5). A "little Hitler" might even become a center of positive creativity, ratifying not only the acceptance principle but Fromm's (1973) contention that the worst destructiveness often follows from frustrated creativity.

Another obstacle to implementing the acceptance principle is its abuse by today's pop therapy cults, which have become like religions in their own right, often without a god and producing less than desirable results. The pop therapy premise, an outgrowth of nineteenth century Romanticism, seems to be that the "OKness of human potential" can fully flower only when free of restrictive sociopolitical or theological limitations. If we experience ourselves fully, "flow with it," "let it happen," express our feelings fully, then all will be well.

Current statistics hardly bear out this claim — for crime and terrorism, alienation in human relationships, escapism through drug abuse and suicide, as well as our political-economic quagmire. Yet a large segment of our society finds it difficult to reject these premises. To make matters worse, there is a striking yet superficial similarity between this "pop ethic" and the affect-containment strategies that are otherwise so powerful.

Pop therapy has missed the point. We do not need to be free of such limitations in order to live fully — it is quite the reverse. To repudiate all restrictive limits, values, discipline, and structure is to repudiate civilization, and paradoxically this outright rejection can become our ball and chain. In this case what is most liberating is freedom *from the need to be liberated*. Under the seductive word "liberation," pop therapy's proponents had learned a subtle nonacceptance: repudiation of certain basics that are required for organized cooperative adult living. Accepting these basic limitations, commitments, and responsibilities paradoxically liberates us.

In principle, nonacceptance should apply only to actions or behaviors deemed evil, while accepting all that actually exists. In practice, it is not always possible, nor necessarily always desirable. To a degree, a certain amount of struggle to mold that which is into what "should be" may provide much of life's creative force. Nonacceptance may extend beyond the specificity of evil behavior to the point of constituting a principle of its own, just as necessary for healthy living as faithful acceptance of self and others. A balance of the two opposites is required, coexisting in a creative tension that no scientific principles can resolve.

Existential nonacceptance or nonacceptance of basic being is probably healthy in two respects: 1) boundary setting, or the process of defining who we are by excluding what we are *not*, and 2) the formation of an ideal self-image, or what "should be," that can guide our creative strivings even while interfering with faithful acceptance of what actually is.

More than we like to realize, maturation, self-identity, power, and sense of direction require a process of *excluding* important potentials. Choosing a career means rejecting a hundred others. Defining what we stand for means excluding what we do not, and what we reject is often as valid as what we choose; yet without such a choice we may remain infantile. Pride in "open-mindedness" can sometimes be a cop-out for refusal to mature. Thus, failure to forcefully create and direct our own "reality" is failure to assume the joys as well as the burdens of adult living.

The formation of an ideal self-image, or what "should be," is more problematic. The negative aspects of this process are well known and may be referred to as *pride* or its psychiatric equivalent, *narcissism*. Such a negative connotation fails to take into account the importance of a self-image in shaping our sense of direction. Of recent experts on narcissism, only Kohut (1966, 1977) has promoted its cause as essential to all human living, undergoing a development parallel with that of object relations, one reinforcing the other. Piaget, as interpreted by

Flavell (1963), points out that *all human knowledge is the formation and manipulation of internal images* that correspond to external reality in a way that helps us guide our lives, but that should not be mistaken for the reality itself. All images must be contrasted with the "really real", yet all are essential to life. The classic tragedy of human life is to live for the sake of some abstract ideal image of self, others, and reality that never was, is not, and never can be. Real living then gets lost in the shuffle. "False self" is mistaken for true self; instead of reality there is only a utopian image. Narcissism probably becomes pathological only when the patient is unable to distinguish his image from what is "really real." The image here becomes *his* reality. To reclaim health a narcissistic patient must often give up his images with all of their consolation as well as limitation, often only with a bitter struggle, pain, and overwhelming grief.

Healthy self-esteem requires faith and acceptance; identity and power for action requires antifaith and nonacceptance. These principles are continually in dynamic tension with one another, a balance that must be defined individually by every unique human being. Further acceptance/nonacceptance dilemmas are illustrated by another case, Hanging On. Because of their relevance to the broad domain of human life far beyond the psychiatrist's consulting room, they will be brought together again in this book's Epilogue — Faith, Force, and Forgiveness.

CASE 3. WAR VETERAN

A 36-year-old war veteran sought treatment for episodic depressed mood and intense unstable relationships that had often dissolved because of the patient's resorting to physical violence, following which he was contrite, remorseful, and often despondent. He met criteria for a diagnosis of borderline personality; in some ways he was even more disturbed, yet in others, he showed a more healthy core and a good value structure. Reviewing his war experiences provided some but only partial relief.

After considerable exploratory therapy, the focal point proved to be dissection of a recent violent episode. The patient was able to delineate three steps in this internal dialogue: 1) "I'm getting uptight —

this could mean trouble — I don't want there to be trouble"; 2) "You [sic] stupid s[deleted]; you sure are stupid; you're doing it again; what in the hell is the matter with you anyway !@$%#$!#!!!"; and 3) loss of control. Reviewing these steps with the patient clarified that step 1 was entirely appropriate: a concerned awareness of potential trouble and a desire to avert it. The problem was at step 2, the entirely unnecessary negative attribution of his feelings that led to such desperate avoidance behavior that he abdicated control, and the most feared catastrophe became virtually inevitable.

The patient was advised to approach the process on any future occasions as follows: 1) "I am angry; it is all right to feel angry"; 2) "I am and will remain in full control over how I choose to act or not act on that anger"; and 3) by voluntary choice remain in control, having revised step 2 to make this choice feasible. In other words, he needs to upgrade his internal parenting. He briefly reviewed with some sadness how he had never had this parenting in childhood, and what a relief it was to know that it was possible and would work. Several weeks later he and his grateful spouse terminated treatment, reporting a great increase in social and occupational functioning, mood, and closeness. A year later he contacted me reporting a continued growth and an increased satisfaction in healthy living.

CLEARING THE CATEGORIES: JUDGMENTAL ERRORS

Many psychiatric patients viciously denigrate themselves as reprehensible human beings and reject their feelings that they label abnormal, perverse, or otherwise simply bad. At the same time they abdicate control over some truly destructive deeds that "just happen — [they] can't help it." Typical in severe personality disorders, this reduces to a common logical fallacy that value judgments should be placed on one's feelings and basic being rather than on the behaviors or actions to which they properly apply. It is a confusion between the categories of feelings and behaviors.

Feelings are an important aspect of basic being not subject to value judgments — they simply are. The common notion of "good" and "bad" feelings is inappropriate; rather, it should be "pleasant" and "unpleasant." As with War Veteran, negative attribution of feelings and selfhood simply increases the avoidance behavior and makes abdication

of responsibility all the more likely. I formerly referred to this fallacy
as the "judgmental category error, ethical type." It is outlined in Table
3.2, depicting the continuum of basic being, feelings, thoughts, impulses, and finally, behaviors or actions.

Moral judgment is unambiguously appropriate only at the level of
behavior and action; only our overt actions, over which a healthy individual has full voluntary control, directly impact others. The other
end of the continuum, basic being, is least open to such judgment—
it simply is. Feelings are pleasant or unpleasant, not good or bad. As
I often put it to patients, feelings are "not illegal, immoral, or fatal."
One's thoughts and impulses are a gray area, generally dealt with as
feelings and similarly distinguished from behaviors. A thought is "bad"
only when voluntarily choosing to dwell on a negative or vengeful one
results in unpleasant consequences. In this case, its voluntariness and
its measurable consequences lend the thought much of the characteristics of a behavior in itself.

The patient first must distinguish the categories of feelings and actions, eventually enabling the acceptance of feelings. This takes the
pressure off, making it easier to control one's actions. Confident in
his mastery of his actions, a patient then feels safer in accepting his
unpleasant feelings. It is hoped that a beneficent circle will follow.
Whether through experiential affect-containment strategies or their
cognitive equivalent, like War Veteran, clearing the categories is often

TABLE 3.2
Judgmental Categories

	Basic Being*	Acceptance
levels	⌐ Feelings	Acceptance
often		
confused in	Thoughts, Impulses	(grey area)
affective &		
behavior	⌐ Actions, Behaviors	Nonacceptance
disorders		Control
		Moral Judgment

*Basic being is often difficult to distinguish from ideal image or from the collec-
tive of habitual behaviors.

the focal point for personality disorders. The cognitive therapy of Beck (1976) and the rational-emotive therapy of Ellis (1962) also act at this level.

Common psychological variations on this theme are summarized in the words of abuse list presented in Table 3.3 for patients in ongoing psychotherapy. The suggested substitutions have a common goal of

TABLE 3.3
Words of Abuse

Word of Abuse	Corrective Substitute
BUT	And
TRY (a)—as cop-out (e.g., "I'll *try* to clean up my room")	(a)—Will, Won't
(b)—as paradox (e.g., "*Try* to go to sleep quickly!")	(b)—Allow, Permit, Let
SHOULD	Will, Won't Want to, Don't want to
CAN'T	Won't
NEED	Want
GET RID OF	Change, Modify, Outgrow, Integrate
ALWAYS, NEVER	Something not black and white (e.g., "All too often . . . ")
SORRY	I don't want you to be angry with me
IT (where active process is misdescribed as if an entity or thing; e.g., "My 'illness' causes me to . . . ")	Reframe entire sentence in a way that validates self as an active agent
YOU (complex; confusion of self/ other boundaries, attributing to others what applies to self; games, projective identification, mind-reading)	I

changing inappropriate psychological nonacceptance to positive acceptance, containment, and control. At a developmental level, the word of abuse is often a childlike cop-out for responsibility, such as "I'll try" really meaning that "I won't, but I don't want to be held to blame for this obstinacy." Confusion between levels also leads to using a word of abuse (see chapter on multiple consciousness; see also Beahrs, 1982b). "Trying" to go to sleep or to get sexually aroused — attempting to do at the voluntary level what can happen only spontaneously — often leads to failure. Time structure is their opposite; here voluntary action is required and letting it "just happen" leads to failure to organize and to direct one's life in a manner required by adult social living.

An additional treatment dilemma transcends simple acceptance vs. nonacceptance and clear thinking. This is the question of what to do when what is useful clinically conflicts with what is factually true, and the conflict appears irreconcilable. Case 4 presents an individual who remains stuck in his pathological behavior, despite having apparently identified and worked through all of his real issues. The subsequent discussion raises the possibility that deliberately altering the patient's psychological reality might be an option to consider. Relativity of truth and utility is one of the more challenging correlates of uncertainty and will recur at several points in the next two chapters, which continue to elaborate the characteristic of the psychological level.

CASE 4. HANGING ON

Rodney is a 40-year-old man who has carved out an impressive engineering career despite a struggle against continuing self-doubts, inhibitions, and episodic despair. He undergoes wide mood swings and has not responded to biological treatment or exploratory psychotherapy. While his symptoms have not prevented impressive outward success, he is unable to really let go of either the fear of some imaginary catastrophe or of bitterness from multiple early emotional depredations. Exploration has revealed a few early-life traumas, fears of abandonment and annihilation, as well as of engulfment in something "not truly [his]". He cannot fully allow himself the uninhibited joys of adult intimacy or truly appreciate the fruits of his very real success. Life is a constant struggle but what he is struggling for or against is not entirely clear. So far, the case is unresolved. The dilemmas are addressed in the following section.

FATE: TO ACCEPT OR CHANGE?

Freud (1920/1975) explained hanging on to symptoms that already should have resolved as argument for a fundamental "death instinct." It may be an unconscious attempt to gain mastery over an early trauma whose associated suffering would otherwise be unbearable. More recent analysts, e.g., Bellak and Small (1978), explain it more in terms of *multideterminism*: since so many factors contribute to creating the symptom, then no matter what aspect of it is dealt with, some evidence of it will remain.

Goulding and Goulding (1979) would search for this patient's early *life decision*. When identified, the patient would make a "redecision" for healthy living. The Gouldings explicitly state that the patient must give up struggling against a past that cannot be changed and accept the full impact of his tragic history. The patient will fear being overwhelmed by grief, but going through this grief process will liberate him. Lowen (1983) would describe him as hanging on to an ideal self-image that prevents his facing the "true horror" of his life, also advocates stark reality testing, facing the horror and grief, which will set him free. All have in common the necessity of giving up self-images (that which "should be"), grieving, letting go, and then moving ahead.

Pitted against this reasoning is Erickson's fabled case of the February Man (Erickson, 1980, Vol. IV, pp. 525–542). Under skilled hypnotic age regression with subsequent amnesia, a new benevolent parental introject was introduced to a deprived patient at a regressed age of three, a Santa Claus-like figure called the February Man, after the patient's month of birth. Subsequent sessions introduced this figure to the regressed patient at older ages, so that eventually the developing relationship *that never occurred* had been installed as an indelible feature of this patient's "past history." As expected, this patient progressed toward good health.

Freud (1916/1979) noted a difference between a patient's reported psychological history and what really happened, ascertaining that it was adequate for practical purposes to work with the substrate of psychological reality, and that what was "real" is relatively irrelevant.

Berne (1972) emphasized similarly that it was a child's experience and interpretation of parental action that was important, rather than what the parent actually said or did.

The most potent "changing the past" strategy was proposed by Roberts (1974). She describes a "natural hypnosis exercise": the patient simply takes ten minutes a day to imagine reliving his past as he would have liked it to happen, then lets go of the fantasy and continues with his day. The positive effects are expected to occur within a month, as if by themselves—similar to Erickson's February Man. Changing the future is less problematic and employs a similar "point of power exercise": the patient takes ten minutes a day to imagine his activities at some future time as he would like it to be, then lets go of the fantasy. This can help organize his life toward that goal. These are quite similar to Erickson's "time projection" approaches (Beahrs, 1971).

Like the many conundrums that pervade our professional work, far beyond scientific specification, the dilemma of whether to accept one's fate, change it, or both at different levels, including both the psychological past and the future, is one that does not admit of easy resolution. Much more understanding is needed.

CHOICE AND THE FRAME OF REFERENCE

In our daily lives the question is not usually whether to accept or not to accept; rather it is when and where, with whom and in what situation, to what degree and at what level. Few determinants of mental health are more pivotal than what we seek and avoid, reflecting what we accept and do not accept, but the complexities of human motivation must forever transcend precise specification. Multiple nuances of pride and identity, personality quirks, idiosyncratic word connotations, as well as differing value priorities, etc. ensure that "cookbook" answers are not possible. However, two pressing questions demand our attention: 1) How do we define our values, identity, and direction in the light of this uncertainty? and 2) How do we best discuss the patient's problems with him, a separate person whose priorities and connotations are so different from ours that for all practical purposes we speak different languages?

The first question is easier: it is virtually unanswerable, except by choice of the individual involved. With absolute moral dictates limited by the many roots of uncertainty, the best one can do is define his own values and then make his life choices on the basis of a moral presumption, as presented in the Introduction and this chapter's overview. All the psychiatrist can do is deal with the context within which these choices are made. The second question is the most pressing problem that faces every psychotherapist in every new clinical situation: how to determine what the context even is and how to mold it in order to encourage a more positive outcome.

The irony of psychiatric practice is that although it is the patient who is the one seeking change and whose "language" may contain the seeds of his problem, it is the presumably more healthy therapist who must defer and speak the patient's language rather than the patient's speaking his. It is neither fair nor scientific, but is simply the way things work best. To change another person we let him be who he is while changing ourselves, thereby changing the context within which the other person makes his own choices.

To "speak the patient's language" is a hallmark of strategic and Ericksonian approaches, but ultimately is beyond any textbook and part of the skill of living. It boils down to simple human decency and respect for personal boundaries; a therapist can and should change only his own behavior while the patient charts his own course. With disturbed boundaries contributing to much of the most severe psychopathology (see Chapter 4 and Epilogue), this simple clarity of awareness and respect for the patient's dignity may ultimately be what is most curative in good psychotherapy.

4

Control and Face-Saving

OVERVIEW

Control of and by others is one of the most basic as well as most problematic features of the social dimension in human living. It is an essential feature of life. It is impossible not to control and be controlled, just as it is impossible not to communicate (Watzlawick, Beavin, & Jackson, 1967). An element of control is inherent in all communication (Haley, 1963). The question is not whether to control, but how and toward what end. Whatever their cause, many psychiatric disorders can be looked upon as disorders of control: the patient's attempts at controlling his environment are either ineffective, excessive, or misdirected; otherwise he would not be a patient.

The patient employs the psychiatrist to influence him, both to feel better and function better in the social arenas of love and work, which Freud rightly considered the measures of mental health. The bottom line, then, is that the psychiatrist's job is to control. However, there are questions we need to ask about any controlling behavior: first, is the control effective; second, is it desirable, reasonably respectful of other people and their needs as well as one's own; and third, when it is either not effective, undesirable, or both, how can we best influence the situation in a desirable direction?

A psychiatrist in a democratic society must simultaneously meet two often conflicting responsibilities with which he is charged. First, he must effectively control his clientele, or he is not worth his fee.

64

Second, he must respect his patient's autonomy, his separateness as a human being who, by necessity, will have his own likes and dislikes, value priorities, and personal style. He must help the patient achieve an identity true to himself, not to the psychiatrist's ideal image. Every discussion of psychiatric treatment must remain ever-cognizant of these two responsibilities — effectiveness and respect for the patient's autonomy.

Human control can be divided and subdivided in several ways. These generally overlap, and the prevalence of one or more factors is only relative. First, control can be described along the dimensions of active/passive, direct/indirect, and desirable/undesirable. Second are three axes of the biopsychosocial model: medical, developmental, and social. Finally, there are the complex issues of personal boundaries, to which all axes contribute even if psychological development predominates.

Controlling behavior occurs along several overlapping dimensions: active/passive; direct/indirect; and desirable/undesirable. Active control is exemplified by the military commander, who directs his troops' actions and can enforce his commands with severe disciplinary consequences. By contrast, the newborn infant and the infirm control others passively, the very poignancy of their distress and helplessness serving to bend others to their will.

Direct control is "up front": who is doing what to whom and for what purpose is evident to everyone concerned. Indirect control may be equally purposeful (or not) but its aim and method are often unclear and covert. Active control is often direct, as exemplified by the military commander, but may be indirect, as in many Ericksonian treatment strategies. Passive control is often indirect, but may be direct, as in the strategic nonviolence of Ghandi and Martin Luther King. Milton Erickson most clearly recognized the importance of control at both levels. Most people believe that the direct type of control should dominate, at least in an executive role. This value judgment is qualified by an equally pervasive opposite: the recognized need for tact, diplomacy, and "timing," and the need to permit face-saving, all of which are better achieved by optimal indirectness. Like all polar opposites, there can be no absolute guidelines as to what or how much of each is best.

The third dimension of control, whether it is desirable or not, can be determined only by one's value priorities; these are necessarily beyond science. For example, the demand that we respect a patient's autonomy is not shared by all cultures, and is based on mutually agreed-upon foundations of our democratic society. Controversies about human rights pervade psychiatric practice and are often a major determining factor in our choice of treatment strategy.

Adequate ability to control the environment requires an intact body, mature cognitive/behavioral skills, and confidence in one's social network. Impairment at any of these levels can lead to dysfunctional controlling behavior, usually passive. Hence, dysfunctional control can be understood along several axes of the biopsychosocial model that again overlap with one another: The medical axis clarifies that gross impairment of cerebral function from any cause can lead to intractable controlling behavior. The developmental axis understands passive control as infantile behavior arising from failure to develop more active adult coping skills. The social axis reflects the use of psychiatric impairment to control others, what Haley (1963) referred to as "symptoms as power tactics." All of these lead to different formulation and treatment, but rarely does one axis operate independently from the others; which, if any, is primary often remains unclear. Hence, an open-minded eclecticism is essential to evaluating and treating control dilemmas.

When assessing disorders of control, we must continually keep in mind the medical axis. When a physical or mental illness impairs the organism's ability to cope, more recently acquired skills are the first to go, with a patient's control tactics becoming primitive not because of defective development or social stress, but because the higher functions have been assaulted and put out of commission. The most intractable passive controllers in my experience have subsequently been shown to suffer from a clear medical illness: not only process schizophrenia, but hypothyroid, diabetes, pernicious anemia, brain tumor, and Alzheimer's dementia; the final common pathway of all of these conditions can be malignant passive control. If these are dealt with only at the manifest psychosocial level, not only will they resist treatment, but a potentially curable medical condition may go unrecognized, a tragedy that happens all too frequently in our work.

When a patient lacks social confidence or fears retribution for active control strategies, he will usually control others passively, often through use of symptoms. Sometimes this may be direct and intentional, but more often is experienced as illness by the patient. Very Sickest, the first case that will be presented, demonstrates the social axis along with overlapping contributions from the medical. The developmental axis is more difficult to understand in isolation from the other two, and is best described in terms of disturbed interpersonal boundaries: confusion as to who can and should do what to whom.

Boundary problems occur at three levels: delusions of control, projective identification, and ulterior transactions or psychological games. Delusions of control are the most severe and include ideas of thought broadcasting, thought insertion, and thought withdrawal, hallmarks of the schizophrenic process. Often a result of biological derangement — thus the medical axis — these frequently respond to thought-organizing antipsychotic medication. An in-between type of boundary confusion is referred to as projective identification, a common manifestation in those patients who require long-term psychotherapy. In psychological games (Berne, 1964), the ulterior motive usually determines the outcome of a complex transaction, and can be seen as an awkward attempt to reassert autonomy otherwise disowned. Most game "antitheses" simply force the more appropriate reassertion of personal boundaries.

Just as the roots of dysfunctional control are complex and manifold, so is its treatment. To modify aberrant controlling behavior requires an eclectic approach that encompasses almost the entire therapeutic armamentarium of the mental health profession. When dysfunctional control is deemed to be the primary target of intervention, we need to make yet a further distinction — whether it is limited to a few specific behaviors or pervades almost the patient's entire personality.

Where the control is specific, circumscribed, and focal, the strategic therapies derived from hypnosis are the most potent and respectful techniques for modifying it. When pervasive control issues dominate the clinical picture at many levels, either of two nearly opposite strategies may be needed: first, refusal to treat the patient at all or redefine treatment goals, such as limiting the patient's expectations; second, when treatment is attempted, both patient and therapist must be prepared for it to be comprehensive and long-term. Regressive dependency is a serious concern in these cases, with the therapist often walking a tightrope between fostering and limiting this dependency. This requires all of the skill and finesse that only extended training and supervision can provide.

Last to be discussed, but one of the most important intangibles, is the all-pervasive human need to save face. Psychiatrists have long been trained to look for and confront unconscious resistance to treatment, but more recent hypnotic data (Beahrs, 1982a; LeCron, 1970) suggests that resistance may arise just as much at the executive or conscious level. It is often based on the "irrational inviolables" that contribute to pride and sense of identity. These demand the respect of the therapist, and are only beginning to be addressed by our profession. "Creative face-saving" is a whole new vista for psychiatric study that this awareness opens to our view.

CASE 1. THE VERY SICKEST: FLORID PASSIVE CONTROL

Mrs. C was a 60-year-old woman whose twenty-five years of marriage were burdened by a variety of florid and incapacitating psychiatric symptoms. Initially depressive, the patient had made several near-lethal suicide attempts early in this course, and was hospitalized for prolonged periods of time with a diagnosis of psychotic depression. On other occasions she had been frankly psychotic, talking desperately about a variety of various plots, others passing surveillance upon her, and her needing to save the world from its own sins. Diagnoses have included psychotic depression, schizophrenia, and atypical bipolar disorder. She did not respond well to antipsychotic medication, antidepressants, or lithium, and ECT resulted in only transient relief.

It was not clear in her initial visit why she was seeking my help. However, during history taking she became visibly dysphoric, with rapid strained respiration, moaning and whining, expressing her agony in colorful descriptions, and chants of "I am just so sick — nothing I can do — *so sick!*" Hardly a word could be squeezed in edgewise. Sensing a need to take charge, I simply asked her to sit quietly, close her eyes, and feel her feelings as *intensely as she possibly could* for a full five minutes. "Oh, God, no, doctor! Please — anything but that!" Firmly holding her to her assigned task, essentially an emergency awareness induction (see Chapter 3, pp. 49–50), led to transient relief and partial completion of a psychiatric history taking: Essential features were a colorful personality style with entirely intact cognitive function and reality testing, a history of refractory dysphoric symptoms, and presence of a dutiful husband who both loved his wife deeply and never challenged his duty to see her through her misery, despite being paralyzed with exasperation. A contract for ongoing treatment was arranged.

Not long thereafter I was notified that Mrs. C had been hospitalized in the county holding unit for "desperation." On my first visit with her she sang her "*so sick*" chant. Attempting both to speak her language and to take charge, I assumed the manner of an old-style benevolent authoritarian physician, and gave her a pronouncement: She was indeed sick, *very* sick, one of the sickest people I have ever had to treat. But I was not sure if she was as sick as she *needed* to be. Had she heard the old cliché that "one must get sicker before one can truly get well?" Yes, she had. Then she was under doctor's orders to do that *right now*, in the safety of the hospital setting. As soon as possible, she was to make herself the *sickest* person on the ward! "I'll try [gasp, wheeze] I'll try."

After several days, nursing staff welcomed me on morning rounds with the information that Mrs. C was too sick to get out of bed. "Ohhh, it's all over — it's no use trying anymore — I might as well give up and die [moan, whimper]." After respectfully complimenting her on the quality of her sickness, I nonetheless called her attention to a regressed schizophrenic who was huddled in a corner: "Look, there is someone even sicker than you. You're not doing your job — you better get with it!" She again assured me that she would try.

Showing up for ward rounds the next morning, I was met inside the door by Mrs. C, who was nattily dressed up in a business suit and carrying a packed suitcase. "*Doctor* Beahrs, I am sick and tired of all this bullshit! This place is only for crazies, and I'm going to leave right now and start living!!" Commenting only that she appeared better and probably did not meet criteria for involuntary commitment, I respected her right to go home but cautioned her about whether or not she was getting well "too soon." Arrangements for ongoing outpatient treatment were agreed upon. Following discharge Mrs. C kept regular appointments with me and was usually accompanied by her dutiful husband. Her colorful personality had become more consistently manifest, and she confronted her husband with a variety of old and current transgressions, some real and some highly exaggerated. With delight, her husband joined the fray.

Of further interest, a glucose tolerance test revealed a markedly abnormal pattern, with a rapid pc rise in blood glucose to nearly 300 mg %, followed by a drop to nearly 30 accompanied by adrenergic symptoms: borderline diabetes with reactive hypoglycemia. The patient was placed on a modified diabetic diet. Her only subsequent hospitalization was for a brief psychotic episode after she became intoxicated at a party.

PASSIVE CONTROL

The need to be in control and to control others should not always call to mind psychopathology. It is a basic function of all human living and probably of the entire animal kingdom. An infant is born helpless and much of the maturation process can be considered as learning to actively control the environment and take care of one's self, instead of depending upon the needs and whims of others. Terr's (1983) study of traumatized children showed that nothing is more devastating to a growing child than to feel utterly helpless in the face of some malevolent external force. Survivors of combat disasters report similarly and almost invariably manifest a greater need to control and be in control than others. Narcissistic individuals attempt to control other people to support their ideal self-image (Lowen, 1983), while obsessionals control others to protect themselves from *being* controlled. Where normal leaves off and pathology begins is a blurred boundary, depending largely on the extent to which the characteristic interferes with social and occupational functioning. Even passive control is not necessarily unhealthy, as evidenced by the willful disobedience of Ghandi and other civil rightists.

Strategic Psychotherapy

The overall psychotherapeutic strategy is to respect the need for control, define it positively, and in the process to subtly direct it in a manner that is more satisfactory to the patient and his environment. There is no format more effective or suitable for this purpose than the *strategic therapy* format as outlined in the collective works of Erickson (Rossi, 1980), Haley (1963), Watzlawick, Weakland, and Fisch (1974), and Weeks and L'Abate (1982). This is no more than an exercise in clear thinking: First define the problem in clear operational terms, including *how* and in what way it is a problem; describe the attempted solutions employed by patient and significant others and how these have either failed to solve, actually worsened, or might *actually be* the problem; clearly define the goals and formulate a strategy, usually to interdict the attempted solutions; and frame the strategy in terms of the patient's known "language." The overriding concept of positive reframing has already been discussed in depth in Chapter 3, along with the need to "speak the patient's language."

Reverse psychology is only one way of looking at the successful treatment of a case such as Mrs. C. Another is that the pathology has arisen from fighting off certain otherwise healthy feelings as opposed to accepting them, thereby blocking the flow and acting almost like a dam on a river (Beahrs & Humiston, 1974). A third follows from the notion of co-consciousness: a paradoxical directive speaks to important parts of the self not on the surface but with their own conscious needs. For Mrs. C, these included the need to be competitive (the "sick*est*"), to be nurtured and taken care of (to take on the sick role), as well as to be in charge (to *voluntarily* exaggerate her condition). The only thing that is paradoxical in such an approach is that it is *unconventional*.

Supporting the Network

Not all passively controlling patients respond as well to an individually directed strategic approach as Mrs. C did. Some schizophrenics display sufficient impairment to endanger their health and exasperate their relatives, but almost never qualify for involuntary commitment. It almost seems as if they are deliberately employing a type of malignant passive control against their social network for reasons that remain obscure. When such patients refuse help and are not committable, we can work only with their friends and relatives, the support network. Common in mental health center practice, the usual approach is to encourage the other individuals to live their own lives and refuse to be controlled by the patient. This can sometimes mean allowing the patient to sleep in the street if, for example, he shows up drunk and psychotic at two in the morning after refusing to keep an appointment and take medication the week before. Work with Mrs. C's husband was an important factor in her treatment as well, though fortunately she was an active participant.

Sometimes it is necessary to seek expert opinion from a third party, usually an independent psychiatric consultant. This can often be an effective strategy with very difficult, passively controlling patients.

The consultant makes a strong intervention and assumes the "bad guy" role, permitting treatment with the primary therapist to move ahead.

Supporting Medical Health

We have not yet mentioned the possible role of Mrs. C's diabetes with reactive hypoglycemia. Psychological treatment, which was already well under way, brought considerable improvement before the diagnosis was made and nutritional therapy instituted. The rehospitalization followed and almost certainly resulted from an isolated alcoholic debauchery. Simultaneous use of nutritional management and psychotherapy make it impossible to tease out the relative benefits she would have achieved from each alone. Therefore we do not know the full impact of her medical status.

More significant is the principle. Of the eight passively controlling patients whose behavior appeared most malignant, skillful, and refractory to intervention, seven had a severe medical impairment, definable either at the time or *ex post facto*. One patient almost identical to Mrs. C, except for more stubborn obsessive and paranoid symptoms, was evaluated and given a clean bill of health by a neurologist only one day prior to hospitalization, and six months later was dead of a brain tumor. Another was anemic, with a hemoglobin level lower than 10. Passively controlling behavior resolved almost entirely after he received two units of blood, given against the advice of an internist who said there were not adequate medical indications for the transfusion. Two proved to have myxedema, two Alzheimer's disease, and another pernicious anemia.

To understand the medical axis of passive control is simple if we see control as one of the most basic human needs. Any physical or psychological impairment reduces a person's ability to actively control himself and his environment, increasing the sense of helplessness, which may be mankind's greatest vulnerability. Desperate attempts to control are then simple commonsense psychology. That the techniques employed are passive rather than active follows from the impairment itself. Most striking clinically is the degree of *skill* with which the passive control is often implemented by such patients, which can blur awareness of the extent of their actual disability. With schizophrenia being increasingly understood as an impairment with pronounced biological roots, this line of reasoning probably also applies to these patients as well.

Perhaps nowhere else in psychiatry is an *eclectic* approach so critical, because the many biological, psychological, and social factors that lead to passive control is as great as the multiple etiologies of mental illness itself. Every psychiatrist and psychotherapist should be familiar, if not skilled, with the following measures sometimes employed: symptom prescription (the strategic format), interpretation of resistance, therapeutic double binds, *identifying* with the resistance (as in Gestalt techniques), hypnotic work, confrontation, reframing, game analysis, family therapy, reinforcing the environmental support networks, assiduous protection of the therapist's own professional space, brute force (where criminal activity is involved or patient meets criteria for involuntary commitment), outside consultation, overall *medical* support when indicated, and maximal maintenance of overall health even when no medical pathology is found.

The case of Mrs. C and the subsequent discussion illustrate the importance of the social axis at both the psychological and social levels, as well as the medical axis. The role of the developmental axis could only be speculated upon. But not all passively controlling patients can be treated with such specific approaches.

When control issues pervade nearly the entire personality, as in personality disorders and some neuroses, targets for specific strategic interventions become less clear-cut. We may be faced with a choice between two nearly opposite strategies. First, we can refuse to treat the patient at all, framing this as minding our own business and respecting his autonomy. If we do decide to treat, however, we must be prepared for this treatment to become complex and multifaceted. One of the long-term psychotherapies originally derived from psychoanalysis becomes the primary vehicle in most such cases. Both strategies clarify the importance of the developmental axis and personal boundaries, and are illustrated in the next two cases.

CASE 2. HOPELESS CASE

Mr. Z sought help for dysphoric feelings and incapacities that were never entirely clear. He reported a history of unsuccessful treatments with many therapists using varied techniques and approaches. Beneath the glowing accounts of how his prior therapists had failed was the implicit challenge, "Do you think *you* can help me?" Repetition of this pattern was guaranteed when I responded affirmatively, a trap that many eager and somewhat cocky young therapists fall into, liking to believe that they could attribute the prior treatment failures to the inadequate theory or technique of the prior therapist. The patient had created one difficult situation after another. All of them were dealt with skillfully at first, but the patient's demands escalated and discontent grew exponentially, until the treatment situation became untenable.

Outside consultation was obtained at that point. The patient was confronted with his game of "Help Me But I Won't Let You" (Watzlawick, Weakland, & Fisch, 1974, p. 138). Psychotherapy was described as an inappropriate violation of his autonomy, and it was agreed that treatment should be terminated, that the patient and only the patient could decide how to live his own life, and that no other therapist should even try. Mr. Z continued to seek treatment elsewhere, continuing his pattern.

BOUNDARY PROBLEMS

At first glance it is hard not to attribute maliciousness to a patient such as Mr. Z, who almost anyone can tell has the basic equipment to live healthfully, and not only chooses otherwise, but defeats the most skilled professional attempts to help. A more accurate and less pejorative formulation is one that is compatible with psychoanalytic understanding of borderline and narcissistic personalities (Kernberg, 1975; Masterson, 1981). These patients are felt to have suffered developmental arrest at the toddler stage, when conflicts between dependency and autonomy dominate the growing child's struggles. Similar conflicts are seen also in patients who have suffered gross psychiatric trauma at a later age, due to the debilitating effect of traumatic helplessness.

Such a patient lives and breathes *incongruity*: virtually insatiable dependency needs are pitted against an inviolable demand for autonomy. When he gratifies his need to be taken care of, that part of himself that demands autonomy rightfully perceives the dependency as a threat. This leads to anxiety, which increases the dependency needs. When those are further gratified this increases the anxiety. An escalating vicious circle is created. The resistant treatment-defeating behavior that follows can be conceived of as a misdirected attempt at asserting the autonomy that he had inappropriately given away. Both dependency and autonomy needs are felt with the full force of the survival instinct, which gives the entire complex set of transactions its desperate intensity.

The cognitive component of what I term "Help Me But I Won't Help You" is confusion of interpersonal *boundaries* — failure on the patient's part to recognize who does what to or for whom, who is responsible for what, etc. He attempts to make a therapist responsible for what only he can do for himself, and then rebels against the other person's controlling behavior that was never truly there in the first place.

Such confusion of self and other is characteristic of psychological games, as described by Berne (1964). As Berne defined it, "a game is an ongoing series of complementary ulterior transactions progressing to a well-defined, predictable outcome" (p. 48). One message occurs at the overtly conscious or "social" level, and another at a covert "psychological" level out of the person's usual conscious awareness. The covert transaction eventually gains dominance over the overt one, leading to a "switch" and unpleasant "payoff." Antitheses can be linked together under the overall rubric of *asserting proper boundaries*. In the case of "Why Don't You, Yes But" it is simply refusing to give advice, turning the problem back on the patient with a query such as "My, that is a difficult problem; what *are* you going to do about it?" (Berne, 1964, p. 120). For some patients like Mr. Z the antithesis simply may be "no treatment as the treatment of choice" (Frances, Clarkin, & Perry, 1984a).

Therapist defeaters are clearly described by Watzlawick, Weakland, and Fisch (1974), whose recommended strategy is to reframe our usual "How can I help you?" to "Your situation is hopeless." This leaves the patient "with only two alternatives: either to relinquish his game altogether or to continue it — which he can do only by defeating the expert through proving that improvement *is* possible. In either case the intervention leads to a second-order change" (p. 139). These strategies have in common the theme of *clarifying the interpersonal boundary between the patient and the therapist* — who is responsible for what. Only the patient can make his own decisions and implement them. The therapist can only give of his time and do whatever specific interventions he deems appropriate, and fall within the legal and ethical bounds of his profession. He cannot make the patient into a different person and he should not try.

Many variants of the "hopeless case" technique can be employed within an otherwise satisfactory therapeutic relationship. One is simply to ask the patient if he *believes* he is a hopeless case, or upon what factors his prognosis depends. This may invite discussion of his worst fears, and in turn, motivate him to modify exaggerated prognostic factors that are more under his control than he believed.

I often employ another variant with people seeking treatment for habit disorders. When the initial request is framed as "make me stop smoking," carrying an implied "but I won't let you," I may respond with an unexpected literal truth: "I *can't make* you stop smoking" and follow this with "*I wouldn't even if I could* . . ." With the patient now in a state of alert expectancy, I continue " . . . because that would violate your own birthright of being an autonomous human being, able to make free choices and live with their consequences." Treatment is often quite productive after this initial boundary setting, which is best done at the very first visit.

Boundary confusion occurs at least at three different developmental levels. Psychological games such as those of Mr. Z represent the highest or *neurotic* level, where the patient expresses *conflict* within an otherwise intact sense of self. The most severely disturbed or *psychotic* level includes such symptoms as delusions of thought broadcasting, thought insertion, and thought control, which some consider to be the essence of the schizophrenic process. These are now felt to be biological in origin in the majority of these cases, and they respond better to antipsychotic medication, simple environmental manipulation, and supportive psychotherapy.

Projective identification, the middle level, is a hallmark of borderline personality disorders (Masterson, 1981) and possibly more common in everyday living than formerly has been thought. It will be discussed in more depth following the presentation of Case 3, along with the related issue of regressive dependency.

CASE 3. ANALYSIS INTERMINABLE

Mr. S was a successful 30-year-old married professional who entered formal psychoanalysis for the threefold goal of relieving episodic stress symptoms, achieving more satisfying personal relationships, and developing an in-depth understanding of the human mind using his own as a laboratory. Despite the analyst's characteristic behavioral neutrality, the patient attributed to him an insidious need to control the patient and mold him into something other than what he really was. A *transference neurosis* (Freud, 1916/1979) had emerged, which would now serve the function of allowing him to work through repressed childhood conflicts.

The patient's excessive need to control and avoid being controlled could now be considered as reenactment of his childhood need to avoid terrifying helplessness. His desire for complete intellectual self-understanding was an equivalent way to cope with the uncertainty of life. (Thus, even part of his motive for entering analysis was now suspect.) When the patient actively resisted the direction of treatment because of his fear of being remolded, this was simply a sign that the analysis was going well, since a fundamental vehicle for therapeutic change is the "working through" of resistance.

As time progressed, the situation hardly changed. The patient asserted his autonomy by attempting to drop out of analysis, but this was defined as avoidance or "flight into health." Continuing control struggles as manifested in the transference reflected the obvious persistence of his underlying dynamics. As more years went by, there were additional complications: The financial load was putting a strain on his otherwise adequate marriage and growing family. This exacerbated his previously less severe dysfunctional patterns of coping with relationships. The idea that the whole enterprise might have been a mistake retreated further and further from his mind; the thought that the massive investment of time, money, and emotional stress might have been wasted would have been an intolerable burden to shoulder. Mr. S continues in treatment, far more symptomatic now than he ever had been prior to undertaking the venture. What the end result will be only time can tell.

A GAME WITHOUT END

Psychoanalysis is more vulnerable than most long-term psychotherapy to a self-perpetuating game without end because of the deliberate lack of feedback provided by the analyst. Corrective information is the

antidote to circular reasoning (see Chapter 6), and the very structure
of the analytic situation is intended to prevent that exchange. By
frustrating his ability to play his usual relationship games, the patient
unavoidably regresses to more primitive coping techniques that are
then dealt with. Alternatively framed, in the absence of any real knowledge about the analyst as a person, the patient has no recourse but
to project primitive beliefs he had regarding authority figures in his
early life. This leads to the transference, whereby the hidden (repressed) past becomes manifest in the disguised form of the present
therapeutic relationship, and when the resulting conflicts are addressed
and resolved the original neurosis is gone as well.

Freud (1916/1979) recommended psychoanalysis only for healthy
individuals or those no more disturbed than at the neurotic level —
those with intact sense of self and others. But following the lead of
Kohut (1971), psychoanalysis increasingly has been applied to the narcissistic and borderline personality disorders, and for some it is their
treatment of choice. To avoid a game without end requires some
modification of traditional technique, especially providing information and limits that protect the patient's sense of his own autonomous
boundaries. Confusion of interpersonal boundaries is a crucial factor that differentiates these patients from Freud's classic case load, and
this awareness helps us understand the dilemma of patients like Mr.
Z and Mr. S.

Since the boundaries that define his sense of self and others are in-
secure and threatened, Mr. S does not clearly perceive what belongs
to whom. He then projects his own primitive anxiety into the void
created by the analyst's blank screen. He *experiences* the analyst's *actually having* those feelings: the need to control the patient and rebuild
him according to his own image.

The patient has given the analyst power that he cannot have and
struggles against this, but is prevented from access to the corrective
information that would resolve the problem, leading to a game without
end. What was supposed to be curative instead perpetuates the problem; the attempted solution has *become* the problem.

If the patient's demand for autonomy overpowers both the dependency needs and other problems that led to the therapy, the patient will
probably break off analysis and the traumatic unresolved transference
may become walled off. If a patient's sense of OKness is more depend-

ent on external support, however, the patient will await this permission from the therapist, and such feedback is exactly what the analyst will not do by the very definition of the analytic situation.

This is not the only paradox in psychoanalysis. Its nondirective quality is intended to respect autonomy, but it is only by virtue of the intensity of treatment in frequency and time that it is even possible for the therapist to mold the patient into something other than what he really is, Mr. S's worst fear. Even though the original boundary error was of the patient's choice, subsequent transactions then give it real substance. The analyst cannot help imposing his own values by such subtle conditioning reinforcement as the timing of "um-hums" (Dollard & Miller, 1950).

While psychoanalysis is often considered the only vehicle for complete self-knowledge, this knowledge is equally altered by that very same subtle intrusion of the analyst's beliefs and values. Perhaps a disciplined regimen of autohypnotic self-exploration à la LeCron (1964/ 1970) is more intellectually pure by very virtue of its *lack* of an outside therapist. But this does not take into account that central aspect of Mr. S's psychodynamics that led to the game without end in the first place. This is projective identification, a type of boundary confusion probably much more common in most human life than has been recognized.

PROJECTIVE IDENTIFICATION AND
REGRESSIVE DEPENDENCY

By projective identification I refer to a process by which an individual experiences his thoughts, feelings, and impulses as though they were what a significant other person were thinking and feeling, and then attempts to control in the other person what was never true of that person in the first place. In an individual with otherwise intact reality testing, the patient actually *perceives* that the other person is feeling what only the patient is feeling. This perception carries the veracity of eyewitness testimony, i.e., "I saw it with my own eyes." Seeing is believing, which leads to defensive behavior that often provokes others to actually feel in the ways that the patient had attributed, reinforcing the patient's original misperception and creating a vicious circle.

This problem may be a fundamental root of the current instability of marriage, correlating with the frequency of personality disorders in our time compared to Freud's. One can only imagine the exasperation of being continually "projectively identified upon" by one's spouse. Again, the results may perpetuate the cause in much the manner of a vicious circle, thus being a problem of the gravest social import.

For a patient in treatment, almost any action may have undesirable consequences if this fundamental disorder of boundaries is not resolved. Breaking off analysis may lead to defensive avoidance of unresolved transference, but continuing for the therapist's approval is to invite interminable analysis. Because the perceived boundary confusion is so pervasive, intense, and subjectively real, I cannot imagine any brief strategic approach being definitive. I have found none in either my own clinical experience or the literature.

However, there is a strategy: to point the patient's awareness toward the developmental origin of his dysphoria, taking the pressure off his current real-life associates. But this must be repeated over and over and over again, in many different permutations and combinations, a process known as *working through*. Paradoxically, the patients who are most vulnerable to a game without end are the patients who need analysis the very most; if not formal psychoanalysis, at least some variant such as the techniques of Kohut (1977), the more intensive psychotherapies derived from transactional analysis (Haykin, 1980), or body awareness work like Lowen's (1983).

"Regressive dependency" is the increasingly dependent relationship that a patient may form with his therapist or even the entire health care system, accompanied by increasingly primitive maladaptive coping techniques that undermine healthy autonomy in favor of excessive dependency. It is another correlate of boundary confusion and the most serious potential side effect of long-term therapy. In my opinion, it is sufficiently problematic that it should be permitted in the therapeutic situation only when there is no other technique that will be more effective or efficient, or when it occurs anyway despite all reasonable attempts to prevent it. I have found escalating spirals of regressive dependency to occur primarily in three situations, which may overlap. The first refers to a particular type of therapeutic approach, the second to a common type of miscommunication, and the third to the type of patient who is most vulnerable to developing this problem. The first was reviewed in Chapter 3: cathartic, or "get rid of," approaches.

Value judgments against normal uncomfortable feelings can lead to a malignant vicious circle of transient relief followed by yet greater dysphoria, with disintegration of a person's entire personality structure. The corrective is inherent in the attitude one should take toward feelings: to accept and integrate them rather than try to get rid of an important part of one's basic being.

A second root of regressive dependency, usually in a milder form, is a patient's reaction to inappropriate formulations presented by a therapist within an otherwise strong treatment relationship. Here, regressive symptoms are more often a patient's way of indirectly yelling at the therapist to "get off your high horse and see me as I really am!" But for Mr. S, who he "really is" is not clear.

This leads to the third situation, in which those with boundary problems associated with personality disorder create a vicious cycle of projecting responsibility onto the therapist, and then rebelling against it. This is based not on simple dependency, but arises from the incongruity of virtually insatiable dependency needs pitted against a demand for autonomy that is inviolable. With these patients some degree of regressive dependency and its working through may be the only vehicle that can lead to lasting change. The main problem in regressive dependency is its cost in time, money, and emotional stress. If there is an alternate approach, the latter should take priority; if not, we then make the most of what we've got.

This third group of patients represent the developmental axis of passive control, failure of the patient to complete the task of separation-individuation required for autonomous action or to adequately define his own boundaries. To facilitate emotional development is the task of the long-term therapist. He must continually walk a fine line between fostering regressive dependency and respecting autonomy, at all times doing his best to minimize the former and maximize the latter, skillfully utilizing all of the primary behaviors that the patient projects into the therapeutic situation, and doing his best to clarify who is responsible for what.

This chapter concludes with a case vignette and discussion that illustrates the importance of permitting a patient to save face.

When patients finally give up their relentless struggle for control in order to get well, it often feels like they have lost something, given up, or suffered defeat. Sometimes a serendipitous face-saver will emerge that allows the patient to bypass this blow to his pride, and allow the many changes to occur more or less as if by themselves. I am encouraging our profession to develop creative face-saving more systematically into our treatment armamentarium.

CASE 4. THE HYPOGLYCEMIC/NONHYPOGLYCEMIC

Mrs. F is a middle-aged housewife who sought psychiatric consultation for increasing depression with inappropriate anxiety attacks and outbursts of irrational rage. Her eating habits were irregular, and she consumed large amounts of coffee, junk food, and occasionally beer and wine. Along with a thorough psychiatric evaluation revealing only minimal evidence of personality disorder, a glucose tolerance test was ordered. It was entirely within normal limits, ruling out hypoglycemia as a diagnosis. But since both her symptoms and eating habits were so similar to those who do have this disorder, I advised the patient to undertake a month's trial of a rigid hypoglycemic-type diet. If she felt and functioned significantly better, this was what mattered the most. She was subsequently lost to follow-up, but I received a grateful correspondence from her many years later sharing her gratitude for my having diagnosed her "hypoglycemia!" She has been nearly asymptomatic since that time, and has been actively attempting to help other individuals with the disorder.

This case demonstrates better than any I know the absurdity of mechanistic causal thinking. Perhaps no one had been helped more by the hypoglycemia concept than this patient, but for no one could that concept have been less true. We can only speculate on the reasons that she got better so quickly; there are many possibilities, and there is no way we can know which, if any, are really accurate. The important thing is that we should not argue with success. Our therapeutic mission is to do whatever is within our power to help a patient get better, and to accomplish this we must work with patients within their own frame of reference and permit them to save face when there is no gross contraindication otherwise.

CREATIVE FACE-SAVING

To get another person to change is seldom easy. But our job is just that, to get another person to accept different beliefs and to modify unacceptable behaviors. To do this it is usually best to let him save face. This is simple commonsense psychology well known to the ancients, and the most important feature of skilled diplomacy. The dearth of professional literature on the topic is perhaps the best testimony to the limits of the purely scientific approach in psychiatry.

Saving face is respecting the self-image that gives a person some sense of personal identity, pride, acceptance, meaning, purpose, and direction. As Carnegie (1936) so aptly put it, it is simply being considerate of another person's feelings. It is human decency to try to change as little as possible in other people, and whenever we must violate that rule to always let the other person save face. This is difficult for the psychiatrist, however, since a patient's self-image often contains the very roots of his pathology. What appears necessary for him to save face may be the opposite of what is necessary to get well.

By virtue of making face-saving more difficult for patients, the "defect" models so prevalent in modern psychiatry make this need more urgent. Psychobiologists know well how much medical noncompliance is due to patients perceiving medication as a constant reminder of their being defective, with its associated sense of shame or loss of face. Much resistance to psychotherapy for personality disorders is similar — the pain of seeing one's self as ever having been defective is unacceptable.

False pride, or *narcissism* in scientific terms, as a root of human evil is a common theme in the history of theology. In tragic literature and opera it is often the vehicle for the inexorable progression of malignant fate (e.g., Verdi & Piave, 1861). What is then needed in these terms, is giving up our narcissistic ideal self-images in order to fulfill our "true self" and get on with the task of living (see especially Chapters 3 and 6; also Kernberg, 1975; Kohut, 1971; Lowen, 1983; Masterson, 1981; Miller, 1979/1981). But why is narcissistic pride so universal and why does simple human decency require that it be respected?

Two perspectives can shed light on the importance of respecting another's pride. First, the narcissistic image appears to be related in some way to maintaining the integrity of our executive function, the still unknown organizing force by which we get our sense of unity in the face of multiplicity, giving stability to our sense of personal identity and a coherent sense of purpose and direction in life. Second, without respecting another's pride, he is likely to resist whatever we attempt as if it were a matter of survival. In a sense it is; if utter helplessness is the most unacceptable of all human feelings, pride is its antithesis, along with the false sense of power that it engenders.

Simple human decency also requires a type of benevolent hypocrisy. In ourselves it is best to ruthlessly confront and often abandon our own false pride, while in others we respect it as if it were a sacred inviolable. Not that this is "right" or "fair"; it is simply the way things work better. We do only what we can do — change ourselves; and we let others be who they are. This respects boundaries and puts the power where it actually is.

The benevolent hypocrisy required for decent living is often reversed in psychiatric practice (see Epilogue). While many patients try to change others' behaviors while treating their own as sacred, violating the rules of decency and perpetuating their own problems, more ironically, the psychiatrist is actually employed to do the very same reversal: to try to make his patient do what only he can do for himself.

The case of the Hypoglycemic/Nonhypoglycemic is an example *par excellence* of creative face-saving. A distinctly neurotic woman was able to reclaim healthy functioning simply by treating a "hypoglycemia" not there by any stretch of the medical imagination. But had this not fortuitously occurred, she probably would have entered long-term psychotherapy and proved most vulnerable to the self-perpetuating games that plagued Analysis Interminable. The dynamics to be addressed would have been most real and the causal implications most relevant. However, it just *worked better* to simply let her be who she is.

The reframing list in Chapter 3 (Table 3.1, p. 46) offers an introduction to techniques for face-saving. A few associated techniques not yet mentioned also apply. Well known to the hypnotist is to *let a little bit of the symptom remain*. If a symptom that the patient is ready to give up is removed by direct suggestion, this usually prevents symptom substitution or other side effects. This suggests that what maintained the symptom may not have been its emotional cathexis as much as the need to save face.

Indirectness is another hallmark of Ericksonian therapy intended to enhance face-saving. It is also described by Carnegie (1936), who says that if it is necessary to criticize someone in the first place, to do it indirectly. Recently, attention has been given to the stories, anecdotes, and metaphors that Erickson often told his patients especially during his late period. These can be curative without the issues ever being brought forward to full consciousness. If the problem can be worked through without the patient even admitting to himself that he has one, this is the ultimate in creative face-saving skill. I often wonder whether the emotional power of tragic literature and opera may arise from their ability to act in this manner: to hold our problems in front of us as if in a mirror, allowing ourselves to make major therapeutic decisions at deep levels while saving face.

5

Multiple

Consciousness

OVERVIEW

This is the first of two chapters that explicitly address the issue of multiplicity on the same broad level. This chapter, continuing the discussion begun in Chapter 3, focuses on the psychological level, defining and developing the implications of the multiple co-conscious mental units or *ego states* that often appear to act independently, and that collectively comprise a person's whole functioning psyche. A corollary theme is the extent to which so many vital aspects of human living can be described only by a tension between polar opposites that cannot be fully resolved and may represent much of the force of life. The next chapter will address the state of our profession at the social level, divided as it must be into multiple competing models, frameworks, and systems, along with the related problem of distinguishing cultism from creativity. As general systems theorists have maintained (Miller & Miller, 1985; von Bertalanffy, 1968; Weiss, 1967), the dilemmas of unity and multiplicity share many common features at whatever level they appear.

The essential theme of the current chapter is that all of the contributions of the last two are relevant not only to the individual as an entity, but to his many separate facets, aspects, or parts, each of which must be considered to some degree as if it were a separate person. Free choice, the acceptance/nonacceptance dilemmas, and the many untestable intangibles in human language remain as important as ever.

But they become even more problematic as we recognize that different parts of an individual may hold different value priorities, maintain different world views, and even speak different languages. In addition, the vicissitudes of active and passive control apply to conflict *within* our psyche as well as conflict between separate individuals and societies. Virtually all the control tactics described in Chapter 4 are employed from time to time by one part-self in an attempt to bend other part-selves or the entire psyche to its will.

The unifying theme is co-consciousness: the simultaneous functioning of the many elements of consciousness within the self proper, each of which has its own relatively separate sense of identity and active experience. The "elements" are what I usually term *ego states*, which Watkins defines as "a coherent system of behaviors and experiences with boundaries more or less permeable which separate it from other such systems within the overall Self" (personal communication, 1979). The ego state concept is similar to that of the intrapsychic system (Grinker, 1975), role (Sarbin & Coe, 1972), and "state of mind" (Horowitz, 1980). Only when the boundaries between such states become overly rigid does an ego state become an "alter-personality," a truly pathological dissociative syndrome (Beahrs, 1982b).

Scientific validation of co-consciousness comes from the hypnosis laboratory (see p. 90). This research shows that co-conscious elements are present throughout hypnotic experience and that hypnosis cannot be separated from nonhypnosis without logical absurdity; hence, co-consciousness must apply to all waking experience.

Implications of co-consciousness extend to the far corners of the mental health profession. For example, the results of a psychological test may depend on what ego state took the test; even those utilizing biological treatment modalities must remain cognizant of the fact that a single intervention may profoundly affect levels of consciousness other than the one that appears to need it. In addition, concepts like *unconscious purpose* and *involuntary action* become relative, since hypnotic inquiry can often identify an ego state that "voluntarily" performed the involuntary action with its own "conscious" purpose, unconscious only from the point of view of the self proper.

Perhaps the paradoxical appeal of psychoanalysis to the scientific bias of our century, despite its overall intangibility, is the respect that it pays to the multidimensional nature of man, which is becoming increasingly clear in the hypnosis laboratory but is not well attended to by hard scientific behaviorism. Freud spoke of "unconscious purpose," revealing his inner awareness that the word *unconscious* connotes much more than simply lack of consciousness. Berne (1961) was clearly aware that his "ego states" were simultaneously present and listening in. Jung (1964) talked of constructs like *anima* and *shadow* as though they were separate personalities. Creative contributors who postulate "parts" of the personality are legion. The point of co-consciousness is that what we formerly referred to as a *psychodynamic mechanism* is no longer some abstract force or drive, but a consciously experiencing entity with which we can and must communicate.

The major clinical implication of co-consciousness is that "others are listening in," and that we should remain aware of saying or doing only what we are willing for everyone present to witness. Paradoxical strategies no longer seem paradoxical if we consider them as direct communication with a part of the person that is hidden but still listening in. If a patient wants to stop smoking but at the same time does not, for example, we may facilitate the therapeutic process by arguing the *disadvantages* of giving up the habit. Taken seriously, the "resistant part" may now become willing to make friends and renegotiate, eventually leading to the desired therapeutic change. Watkins and Watkins (1979b) respect co-consciousness most explicitly with their "ego state therapy" paradigm, or the "use of group and family therapy techniques for the resolution of conflicts between the various ego states that make up a 'family of Self' within a single individual" (p. 184).

Since there is no end to the variety of ways in which different roles and ego states can organize themselves into a functioning psyche, I prefer to avoid overly precise specification of psychodynamic relationships. Rather, I look upon the mind as a symphony orchestra, a complex unity comprising many parts with their own identities, functioning cooperatively under the organizing leadership of an executive, the conductor.

Two questions are posed for further research, in the neurological sciences and in psychology: First, what are the biological mechanisms that might accompany and underlie the dissociative process by which one conscious element is separated from another? Second, and of even greater importance, by what means are our many co-conscious elements organized into a sense of cohesive selfhood? Instead of viewing an illness like multiple personality as a freak of nature, we need to ask the questions, "Why and how does a healthy person have a sense of unity in the face of his multiplicity?" and "Why is it among his most cherished possessions?"

Only then can we begin to obtain greater comprehension of dilemmas like voluntary vs. involuntary action or conscious vs. unconscious experience, since these can have more than a relative validity only when a reference point is clearly defined. If one part lifts the subject's hand but another experiences it as "just happening," our calling the action voluntary depends on whether the first or second part "represents" overall selfhood. Part two is hypnotized and part one is not if we consider involuntariness an important aspect of the hypnotic experience. While science may go far toward answering these vital questions, it must not minimize the significance of the fact that presence of simultaneous opposites pervades human life where it most counts — in our ongoing experience, always the domain to which psychiatrists must attend.

Similar dichotomies abound in human life, the voluntary/involuntary being only the one most clearly associated with multiple consciousness. Others are cooperation/competition; dependency/autonomy, autonomy/intimacy, structure/flexibility, and the faith/antifaith tension described in Chapter 2. Health requires a balance of opposites, each in tension with the other without any guidelines for dictating how much of each or where. With fundamental tension incapable of resolution at the level of human living, scientific precision must necessarily fall short of addressing the human condition.

The simultaneous presence of polar opposites and multiple consciousness together provide the fourth fundamental root of uncertainty in mental health, and the one most clearly characteristic of Heisenberg's uncertainty principle in quantum physics. The latter followed from the dual nature of energy as wave and particle, with the energy of the particle aspect inversely related to the wavelength of the wave aspect: Precision in one measure can be achieved only at the expense of precision in another, overall reliability precluded by the very nature of energy itself.

Following are two extensive discussions regarding current research of co-consciousness, which I believe are needed to establish its current scientific status and to discover how it sometimes goes wrong. The first presents my own understanding of hypnosis research, from which I derive co-consciousness as a fundamental principle of mental functioning. The next section deals with the catastrophic effects of psychological trauma, which are usually dissociative. Then I will illustrate the dilemmas of multiple consciousness with clinical case material, and offer a few simple guidelines for dealing with these troublesome issues in the consulting room. Additional material on ego states as "constructs" will be presented in Chapter 7 in the section on constructs and their limits of reference.

HYPNOSIS AND CO-CONSCIOUSNESS

Validation of multiple consciousness in the normal waking state is based on knowledge of what occurs in the hypnotic state. While few practitioners agree on how hypnosis is best defined, there is still consensus on general features sufficient to establish the study of hypnosis as a scientific discipline. I have incorporated these three features (Beahrs, 1982b, Chapter 2) so that a behavior or an experience is considered hypnotic if it satisfies one or more of the following:

1) *motor* — it is experienced as involuntary, automatic, or spontaneous, as opposed to being done by conscious choice or effort. For example, a hand "just lifts" in a hand levitation;
2) *sensory* — imaginings can be experienced as if actually perceived, enabling all manner of possible distortion in any sensory modality; and
3) *cognitive* — there is a relative increase in magical, symbolic, and pictorial thinking, usually with preservation of reality testing, referred to as "tertiary process" (Arieti, 1976), creativity, or adaptive "regression in the service of the ego" (Gill & Brenman, 1959).

If a subject's behavior and experience are far greater at these three levels than in his usual state of mind, he is said to be in a hypnotic state. Table 5.1 lists the twelve hypnotic phenomena in the Stanford Hypnotic Susceptibility Scale Form C (Weitzenhoffer & Hilgard, 1959) that are typical of the hypnotic state, and all of which can be subsumed in the threefold definition.

A hypnotized subject often shows persisting features different from those of his usual waking state, which leads one to look at it as an

TABLE 5.1
Hypnotizability Norms*

Specific Phenomenon	Subjects Who Respond (%)
MOTOR (Involuntary action)	
hand lowering	92
moving hands apart	88
arm rigidity	45
arm immobilization	36
SENSORY	
mosquito hallucination)eyes closed)	48
taste hallucination	46
anosmia to ammonia	19
hallucinated voice	9
negative visual hallucination (eyes open)	9
COGNITIVE (Regressive)	
dream	44
age regression	43
amnesia	27
Summary	
Easy Motor Items	90
—time distortion in between	
Moderate Depth Hypnotic Items	50
(motor challenge, cognitive-regressive, eyes closed sensory)	
—posthypnotic suggestion and amnesia in between	
Somnambulism	10
(eyes open hallucinations)	

*Data derived from Weitzenhoffer & Hilgard, *Stanford Hypnotic Susceptibility Scale Form C*, Consulting Psychologists Press, Palo Alto, 1959.

altered state or trance. Such characteristics of trance are itemized in Table 5.2. The problem with these models is twofold: few subjects experience all hypnotic phenomena, and trance characteristics are heavily dependent upon the nature of the induction; a subject usually has his own unique profile of hypnotic responses, and he might be deeply hypnotized and still manifest few if any of the classic characteristics of trance.

TABLE 5.2
Characteristics of Trance

EXPRESSION
  immobile, relaxed, less blinking of eyes

SELECTIVE ATTENTION
  rapport
  attention to internal cues
  ideomotor & ideosensory responses

ECONOMY OF MOVEMENT
  catalepsy, time lag
  associated movements

TRANCE LOGIC (Orne, 1959)
  literalness
  tolerance of ambiguity
  symbolism

HYPERSUGGESTIBILITY (Bernheim, 1947)

To understand the implications of hypnosis research for co-consciousness, we need to go back to the banner decade of hypnosis research, the 1970s. The two major trends were the "skeptical" research of T. X. Barber (1972). Sarbin and Coe (1972), and others who claimed that it was meaningless to talk of hypnosis as a special state separate from the continuum of normal waking consciousness; and the "neodissociation" research exemplified by E. R. Hilgard's (1977) discovery of the "hidden observer." Together these constitute a laboratory validation of the necessity of co-consciousness as a feature of normal human consciousness.

The skeptical theorists have demonstrated the ability of variables normally considered nonhypnotic to induce hypnotic trance phenomena (cf. Table 5.3). They reason that virtually all waking procedures are "hypnotic" and that the concept of hypnosis as a *separate state* is therefore unparsimonious, meaningless, and expendable (Barber, 1972). Similarly, it has long been recognized that a subject carrying out a posthypnotic suggestion with amnesia may experience it as having arisen from free choice (nonhypnotic), and give plausible reasons for the "choice" totally unrelated to the hypnosis.

In either case, the boundary between hypnosis and nonhypnosis

TABLE 5.3
Hypnosis-Nonhypnosis Boundary Problems

Nonhypnotic Control Variables as "Hypnotic"
  Imagination (Hilgard, 1968; most others)
  Task motivation (Barber, 1972)
  Relaxation (Edmonston, 1972)
  Role behavior (Sarbin & Coe, 1972)
  Hyperalertness (Barber, 1972)

Hypnotic Behavior as "Nonhypnotic"
  Posthypnotic suggestion with amnesia, experienced and rationalized
    as if freely chosen (common in clinical experience)

---

is blurred. On the one hand, an unfortunate result of this research could be to reject hypnosis altogether as meaningless, so that an increasingly impressive body of hard scientific data would be denied fair hearing by the scientific community. On the other hand, an individual who has experienced or worked with hypnosis and sensed that something very profound was going on is at risk for rejecting the inseparability of hypnosis and nonhypnosis out of hand as contrary to direct observation. And the more one position is maintained, the more vehemently the other is likely to be offered as a "corrective."

Each position misses a vital point resulting in not only the perpetuation of the sorry state of affairs just described, but also the prevention of the so-called skeptical theories from receiving the full scrutiny that they deserve and that could shed much light on the paradoxes inherent in both hypnosis and healthy living. I am referring to a rarely challenged either-or assumption; that is, *either* hypnosis must be an entirely discrete and separable "special state" *or* hypnosis is entirely without meaning.

A far more attractive possibility exists, however, that is both logical and far more able to encompass seemingly contradictory data. This is that we *can* define hypnosis and nonhypnosis in terms of clear operational variables (see Tables 5.2 and 5.3) but that it is not possible to define any particular waking experience as only hypnotic *or* nonhypnotic without some component of the other polarity being present as well. It may be one, the other, and/or both, simultaneously at different levels, similar to the conscious/unconscious dichotomy, which is equally problematic. *Instead of either-or, it may be either-and.* A closer look at this possibility will clarify much of the unity vs. multiplicity dimension with which we are so forcefully faced when presented with a disturbed multiple personality and complex cases like those of Leonard (see p. 103) and Mrs. R.

When a hypnotized subject's hand "just lifts," for example, we can make two assumptions: 1) the "doer" and the "experiencer" must be separate since the latter experiences the former only by its effects; and 2) the "doer" also must be some mental process at a high enough cognitive level to evaluate the hypnotist's communications, decide whether and how to respond to them, and carry out the complex purposeful action required. We usually associate this with consciousness. Only relative to the "experiencer" is the action involuntary, thus, by definition, hypnotic. To the "doer" it is an act of free choice like any other that can be validated by subsequent hypnotic inquiry. We say that this subject is unequivocably hypnotized since his sense of self proper is so closely associated with only the "experiencer." As with the traditional conscious, this is our reference point, and one that eludes current understanding.

Stated more simply, a person's mental status at any given moment will be a gray area, with some characteristics considered hypnotic and others not. For instance, a man driving to the opera with his wife may carry on an in-depth discussion with her of the coming week's plans at a level of deliberation and control that few would call hypnotic. At the same time, the complex, purposeful actions required to drive on a busy freeway "just happen," and the subject might not even remember them after the fact. As the driver he was hypnotized, but as the life planner he was "awake." Even from the reference point of self proper, it is not possible to specify whether the subject was hypnotized or not; he was *both at once.* This is the point of the skeptical theories that is so often missed: It truly is impossible to separate hypnosis from non-hypnosis without logical absurdity, not because the distinctions lack meaning or the definitions are unclear, but because both processes are relevant simultaneously at different levels. Instead of rendering scientific hypnosis meaningless, it demonstrates that what we learn from its study should have equal relevance throughout our general waking experience.

The multiple consciousness implicit in virtually all hypnotic phenomena has become concretized in the laboratory with Hilgard's (1977) discovery of the "hidden observer," which unequivocally extends co-consciousness beyond psychopathology, suggesting that it may be an essential feature of what we refer to as hypnosis. Hilgard also noted a parallel between this phenomenon and the one-way amnesic barrier found in many dual personalities. Watkins and Watkins (1979a) found that different hidden observers could be elicited for different hypnotic states, even in the same normal subject. They were often childlike, had unique personality quirks, and preferred different modes of address. Their more accurate perception was rarely across the board, but more often limited to the test situation from which they had been elicited. They often had a sense of "being there for a reason," and would talk about their purpose in the overall economy of self. Along with some sense of persistence over time, this suggested they may be more than just hypnotic artifacts, perhaps being ongoing components of the subject's psyche that require hypnosis only to be "called forth" or rendered overt. The Watkinses liken them to ego states, or coherent systems of behavior and experience, with more or less permeable boundaries separating them from other such systems within the overall self.

Formal argument is offered elsewhere for co-consciousness as a definitive feature of ongoing human experience, whether hypnotic or not (Beahrs, 1982b, Appendix 1; 1983). This can be approximated by the following syllogism: hidden observers are a rule in hypnosis, derived from empirical evidence; hypnosis cannot be separated from nonhypnosis without logical absurdity—what applies to one must also apply to the other; therefore, hidden observers, and thus co-consciousness, must be the rule for normal human experience as well.

For validation of co-consciousness, one need go no further than the psychiatric consulting room. For example, a patient wants some goal but a symptom contravenes. Later the purpose behind the symptom "comes out" and the patient is now able to tell why he did *not* want the stated goal, and why and how he chose the methods he did to sabotage it. Now out in the open, this contrary motivation most likely had been present all along in similar form, just not openly expressed; it makes more sense of what otherwise would seem unfathomable. A patient's response to a successful confrontation, interpretation, or paradoxical directive also illustrates this concept. The response is often one of positive relief, suggestive of "Wow! Someone finally understands me." Or it could be a fleeting letdown, like "I've been found out; I can't use that rationalization anymore." Both imply more conscious, purposeful imputation than just force or drive. The power of two-chair work and ego-state techniques also suggests that many "drives" reflect consciously experiencing entities that are more than willing to be contacted and given voice (Beahrs & Humiston, 1974).

To assume that "unconscious" processes have their own consciousness can provide a bridge between psychodynamic theory and the indirect approaches of Erickson (Beahrs, 1982a), who defined hypnosis as communication with the unconscious (Beahrs, 1971). Since this implies that it can be contacted with words, the term *unconscious* becomes relative. It would be more accurate to talk about levels of simultaneous consciousness, where one level can be unconscious only relative to another. My "conscious" in the usual psychiatric sense would be whatever is identified as subject or "me" at the moment by whatever carries my experience of "John Beahrsness," my self proper. My "unconscious" can be only what is outside of this; that it has its own conscious experience is not a contradiction, then, but an illustration that consciousness is not either-or but either-*and* at many levels. What self proper is can only be posed for further research.

Pending is the great enigma in co-consciousness: With many persisting ego states at parallel levels of organization, from where do we get our sense of a cohesive self, of being a single mental and physical unit with extension in space and continuity in time? Is there a separate "I" over and above ego states that can decide what role to play at any given moment (Hilgard, 1977) or is self determined only by a hierarchy of competing forces or drives? That it is hard to reduce the executive to a single ego state is evident from a close look at even the P-A-C of Berne (1961). Selfhood or "I-ness" alternates between whichever ego state is executive or running the show, but all the ego states are presumed to be simultaneously conscious; hence, the "I-ness" must be of a different essence. I suspect that we will need to look to the neurological sciences for any resolution of this question.

Neurological study of co-consciousness and the executive function is hampered by the likelihood (Hebb, 1949; Pribram, 1971) that different ego states or thought patterns involve only different patterns of microactivity, each involving the same anatomical structures in a similar way and perhaps using even the same biochemical transmitters. We must then ask: 1) How can two or more complex patterns of activity involving the same structural and chemical pathways be simultaneously active? 2) How are the different patterns (dissociation, stimulus selection) kept separate from one another? and 3) How is only one pattern at a time given access to the motor pathways, enabling it to direct the body's activities, and in some unusual situations having a similar selective access to the mechanisms of allergy? Most important of all, what process *presides* over these others, giving us not only our sense of selfhood but coherence and direction to our life course? Presumptive evidence suggests that the temporal lobes and limbic structures are important for attention and memory, and that biogenic amines play a regulatory role at the chemical level, but more specifics remain only speculative.

TRAUMATIC DISSOCIATION

Multiple consciousness becomes pathological only when it is limited to a rigid repetitive pattern that is maladaptive and interfering with the individual's ability to love and to work. When this is the case, two features stand out: 1) The process is driven by an intensely aversive "traumatic affect" around which the symptoms and signs revolve; and 2) it is accompanied by many phenomena that we have called "hypnotic," occurring beyond the subject's control. Multiple personality disorder (MPD) is a paradigm of spontaneous hypnotic dissociation driven by traumatic affect (Beahrs, 1982b), with similar phenomena having also been noted for phobic and posttraumatic stress disorders (PTSD) (Spiegel, 1984). This twofold process probably applies more broadly than currently recognized, extending to nearly the gamut of those mental disorders with primarily psychological origin.

Two well-recognized aspects of MPD support this twofold process: 1) The pathological split(s) can nearly always be traced back to one or more episodes of gross psychic trauma experienced as a threat to the victim's survival and in the face of which he was *utterly helpless*; 2) almost invariably, such patients are excellent hypnotic subjects. The disorder can even be defined as one of spontaneous hypnosis (Bliss, 1980; Beahrs, 1982b). In the MPD, the primary trauma is usually child abuse, and in PTSD it is either the horror of combat or of natural disasters.

Traumatic affect cannot be defined in terms of familiar emotions like fear, anger, and despair. It is more like a desperate hyperarousal whose intensity and character are overpowering, but which subverts any possibility of effective action. It simply takes over. As a panic attack victim recently described: "I can't even imagine the feeling when it's not there, but when it comes there can be no reasoning—it just takes over wherever I am, whatever I am doing." It is like an imperative to flee, but there is nowhere to go; or to express blind rage, but with no possibility of effective aggression. In any case, it is dysphoric, maximally aversive, and incompatible with normal coping behavior. It is probably the subjective experience of such intense cerebral over-activity that the selective neural activity required for focused problem solving is grossly impaired.

Follow-up studies of traumatized children substantiate the claim that utter helplessness in the face of a catastrophic stressor is the stressor's primary pathogenic feature (Terr, 1983). Four years after the notorious Chowchilla schoolbus kidnapping, 25 children were assessed and contrasted with an otherwise similar control group who had suffered no gross trauma, but only the usual bumps and bruises of everyday living. The traumatized children almost uniformly shared a "mortification regarding (their prior) vulnerability" (p. 1544). Many symptoms were similar to PTSD: cognitive suppression, phobic behavior, denial, and repression.

There was also evidence of spontaneous hypnotic behavior with the type of sensory, volitional, and cognitive distortions that define that state: visualization, displacement of affect, misperception, and time distortion. Over half of the children experienced a "time skew" (p. 1546) in which simple events subsequent to the trauma were falsely "re-membered" as if they had occurred before, and these were then interpreted as if they were a sign to which the child should have paid heed. Nineteen of the 25 (76 percent) believed they had been given such an omen before the kidnapping and that they were therefore to blame for not having taken preventive action. "In a sense, the child chooses personal responsibility and even guilt for the event over utter helplessness and randomness" (p. 1547). More ominous, 23 of the 25 children (92 percent) experienced a sense of foreshortened personal future characteristically absent in the nontraumatized controls. This actually increased over the four-year follow-up period, along with dangerous "post-traumatic play" and other reenactment behavior that again appeared to be an attempt at mastery of the trauma, but which put the children at increased risk of the early demise in which they believed.

In the face of traumatic affect, coping is possible only if some device can be found to set it aside, push it away, or wall it off. This is what spontaneous hypnosis can do, involving as it does some poorly understood ability to separate the "doer" and the "experiencer." Caputo (1977) describes a terrible combat experience when he joined his entire platoon in a wartime atrocity: "Strangest of all had been the sensation of watching myself in a movie. One part of me was doing something while the other part watched from a distance, shocked by the things it saw, yet powerless to stop them from happening" (p. 280).

By a splitting mechanism we do not yet understand, the "doer" could act free of interference from his value system, driven by the force of traumatic affect. The "experiencer" who now provides the retrospective account, was powerless to alter his behavior. Even though its actions were wantonly destructive, the "doer" no longer felt helpless. It was now the "experiencer" who was powerless to stem the inexorable flow of events, even while being shocked and repulsed by what was taking place. It was like he was not himself. He had become two.

The power of traumatic affect both forces the original split and prevents its subsequent resolution, creating a Faustian trade-off illustrated in Figure 5.1. The circle denotes the overall psyche. The "traumatic sector" is that part of the person that experiences the traumatic affect and acts accordingly. It is the part of Caputo that committed the atrocities so unacceptable to his overall values. The conflict-free sector is now able to function free of traumatic interference, which makes it possible to continue going through the motions of life. But this is achieved only at the cost of the problem never being resolved. The many small arrows depict the continuing output of psychic energy required to keep the trauma at bay. The result is the cognitive constriction and blunted affect so characteristic of post-traumatic stress disorder. And the boundary remains sufficiently permeable to permit frequent intrusions of traumatic material into the usual consciousness, such as nightmares and revivifications. The traumatic sector is sufficiently forceful to require phobic avoidance behavior, and sometimes disguised reenactment behavior — such as compulsive rituals and impulsive behaviors — may relieve enough of the pressure to maintain

Figure 5.1. Traumatic dissociation

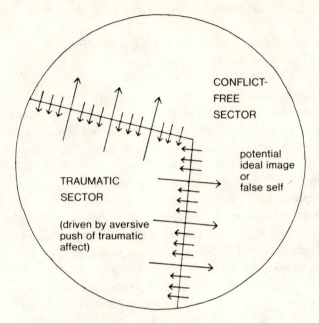

energy expended by conflict-free sector to wall off
(repress) the traumatic sector

intrusions of traumatic material into consciousness

an uneasy balance. As Freud (1916/1979) had long maintained, neurosis is indeed a compromise formation between two opposing forces, each of which is granted only partial expression.

Traumatic dissociation may be equally relevant to the major unresolved dilemma of pathological narcissism. A narcissistic personality may function at a high developmental level in some areas of life, usually educational/occupational, while his impairment in personal relationships may approach psychotic proportions. Masterson (1981) states the dilemma most clearly:

> A controversy has arisen over how to explain that [in] the narcissistic personality disorder . . . a very primitive self-object representation is seen alongside a seemingly high capacity for ego functioning . . . there has yet been no satisfactory resolution of this dilemma either by myself . . . or other authors . . . we hope

in the future to develop a theoretical postulate to resolve this ambiguity. (pp. 11–12)

The mechanism of traumatic dissociation outlined in Figure 5.1 may provide the needed postulate. If the child narcissist-to-be is raised in a sufficiently traumatic environment but has the requisite dissociative ability, he may conveniently "split in two" without fully realizing it. The traumatic sector continues to grapple with his disturbed personal situation, learning unusual coping skills that will not be appropriate in his later adult life while the conflict-free sector addresses such tasks such as school performance. By setting aside the conflict, the conflict-free sector is able to grow and develop, but at the tragic cost that the conflict is never resolved, and perpetuates itself throughout the unfortunate individual's stormy life course.

The conflict-free sector often acquires many characteristics of a "false self," even maintaining its own world view, with values that betray the autonomous self in favor of a well-rationalized effort to keep the trauma at bay. Terr's (1983) research has already shown how one's basic life beliefs are perverted by this post-traumatic process. Carrying most of the person's vital life energy, the split-off traumatic sector binds much of what otherwise would be "true self," but in a limited and circumscribed way that can lead to perverse behavior (Lowen, 1983).

Traumatic dissociation also shares several features with the concept of "life script" developed by Berne (1972); each may lead to belief in a foreshortened personal future, along with specific reckless behaviors likely to fulfill that tragic possibility. It is difficult in such a case to distinguish an automatic response to trauma from a life script consciously chosen by a patient as a child in the face of continuing adversity and limited information. Terr's data demonstrate that attribution of personal responsibility for a trauma can be a defensive avoidance of the helplessness of actual fact, while Berne's TA emphasizes a patient's continuing victim role as a denial of his active role in choosing to at least maintain that role. These perspectives are partly reconciled by David Spiegel's observation (personal communication, 1985) that "the irony is that the PTSD patient truly was helpless at the time of the trauma, but cannot accept that fact. He does not need to be helpless now, but continues to act as though he were a continuing victim of malignant societal forces beyond his control." In either case, the reality of actual fact is denied in a way that perpetuates the symptoms. Where personal responsibility is false but dogmatically maintained, the intriguing possibility emerges that an occasional patient may do better to "own up" to a false responsibility or "script decision" *that never occurred*, only in order to "redecide" in a manner like that suggested by Goulding and Goulding (1979).

When the boundary between two parts of personality becomes overly rigid, these parts may undergo a process of parallel cognitive and emotional development independent of one another. It is then experienced as if the two were truly separate personalities, each with complex integrated behavior patterns and separate social associations. This is the true multiple personality; there is no longer continuity of the self proper. Most commonly the "primary" personality represents the conflict-free sector with its cognitive constriction and blunted affect, and usually maintaining the life position of a victim. The traumatic sector occasionally takes over the body and "comes out," acting in a recklessly destructive manner with tragic consequences.

Intrapsychic trauma proves to be a focal point for many troubled patients. Treatment of post-traumatic stress disorder generally requires that a patient accept his original helplessness in order to reclaim his right to free agency in the here-and-now life situation. A wide variety of treatment strategies are employed, including the affect-containment approaches described in Chapter 3 and multiple-consciousness strategies (see pp. 103–108). When psychological trauma appears to dominate a patient's presenting symptomatology, it is also essential to keep in mind the possibility of false or inappropriate causality. Two possibilities need to be considered here: that focusing upon a traumatic event could be a defensive avoidance of something else or a face-saver. If it is a defensive avoidance, the trauma might well be real but of only secondary importance to another factor. The other factor might be some malignant biological illness whose disruptive effects on brain activity feels like traumatic affect to the patient. Schizophrenia is the example most common in psychiatric work, and to overlook the possibility of neuroleptic medication as the most appropriate focal intervention would be unacceptable. Another factor might be at the social level, with factitious post-traumatic stress being maintained by the patient for clear secondary gain (Sparr & Pankratz, 1983). To save face, some patients talk of trauma in past lives or at birth. If this is not a defensive avoidance of some otherwise available focal point, one may do well to simply work with the patient's presenting frame of reference, as in the case of Hypoglycemic-Nonhypoglycemic in the last chapter.

The following case vignette illustrates the nature of co-consciousness in clinical practice.

CASE 1. LABILE HYPERTENSIVE

Leonard was a 40-year-old male with severe relationship problems, episodic depression complicated by alcohol abuse, and severe hypertensive vascular disease requiring simultaneous treatment with diuretics, beta blockers, and occasionally more potent agents. While discussing his self-destructive behavior there was a twinkle in his eye that made him look like a small child with an ace up his sleeve, quite incongruous with the depressive cast of his overall presentation. It appeared that at least a part of him was enjoying the tragic proceedings. This possibility led me to address that part, which I assumed was most likely there and listening in, even though disowned in the original presentation.

Bitterly resenting the other's placating life position, this formerly disowned part kept trying to "shake some sense" into him and break free. In his usual state, the patient was aware of another persisting state of mind and considered himself to have "two personalities." His usual self was serious and ethical, the other one fun-loving but without limits or true concern for others (cf. "demon," Beahrs, 1982b, Chapters 5–7). Setting the "two" down to the conference table to negotiate led to an appropriate division of roles. The serious part assumed the executive role, providing needed protective structure and just enough discipline to avoid consequences harmful to all concerned. The childlike part was allowed to have fun in a constructive way, contributing life energy to the otherwise depressed executive part.

Following this mediation, his blood pressure returned to the normotensive range, though on medical advice medication was continued to mitigate the expected recurrence of hypertensive episodes. Only diuretics were used. To the amazement of nursing staff, this patient could be persuaded to *purposefully* create a hypertensive episode by simply putting his ego states into conflict, and could equally quickly return it back to the normal range by calling a truce. He could alter his blood pressure by a range of ± 50/20 mm in less than five minutes. sending it up or down at will.

PROBLEM EGO STATES AS A FOCAL POINT

Leonard's case is a classic illustration of the utility of ego state theory, as described by many diverse authorities. His situation closely approximates the Parent-Adult-Child triad of Berne (1961) and the Gestalt model of Perls (1969), but closer yet, the *ego state therapy* model of Watkins and Watkins (1979b). Types of ego states frequently encountered in clinical practice are listed in Table 5.4, while the intricacies and dilemmas of "multiplicity" therapies have been discussed in depth elsewhere (Beahrs, 1982b, Chapters 5–7).

Dealing with a self-defeating ego state may be the focal intervention for many troubled patients. In Leonard's case it was the fun-loving childlike facet of his personality that had flamboyantly sabotaged his overall need for structure and discipline until its own needs were validated. In this case, a workable division of labor was rapidly achieved; it turned the corner for a man with a long history of mixed personality disorder, alcoholism, and hypertension refractory to all interventions previously tried. This illustrates the dynamic of "making friends with demons" (Beahrs, 1982b, Chapter 6); an apparently negative part-self now proved to be the source of much of this patient's vital life energy.

Other self-persecutory ego states seem more like an internal "tyrant" than a mischievous child. Often stubbornly resistant to "making friends" so useful in most childlike states, it attempts to keep the person in what is like a rigid box, fighting off with the full force of the survival instinct any attempts to grow or change. This is the key to the door: The survival element makes sense if a "tyrant" is viewed as an individual's primitive attempt to define his personality structure, his identity as a unique individual that sets him apart from others. To validate this protective function while indirectly suggesting change coupled with face-saving (Chapter 4) may work, but often only after a great struggle. Case 2 in Beahrs (1982b, Chapter 7) also illustrates this process.

Still more difficult and potentially dangerous is an "avenger," an ego state that serves to discharge rage and reap vengeance upon former

TABLE 5.4
Commonly Encountered Ego States

Conscious
  - Primary personality
  - Executive
  - Self 1 (Gallwey, 1976)
  - Conductor

Unconscious
  - Collective of processes leading
    to involuntary or spontaneous action
  - Self 2
  - Orchestra

TA Ego States (Berne, 1961)
  Parent (+) Internal nourishing and limiting functions
          (–) Stifling, indulging
  Adult   (+) Rational problem-solving
          (–) Exclusion of spontaneity
  Child   (+) Life energy basic being
          (–) most problems arising from non-acceptance and lack of control

Common Problems (Beahrs, 1982b)
  Demon   (+) Life energy
          (–) Sabotage, lack of control
  Tyrant (+) Intrapsychic structure
          (–) Self-tyranny
  Avenger (+) original protection in face of helplessness
          (–) Destructiveness
Expansive Ego States
          (+) Creativity, growth
          (–) Psychosis, occult

(+) Coordinating function
    Self identity and outward image
    Time structure
(–) False pride, victim position
    Performance paradoxes
(+) Creativity, spontaneity
    Sleep, sex
    Dreams
    Smooth functioning
(–) multiple problems when beyond awareness and control

Hidden Observers
  (+) Organizing force (?)
      Self-knowledge
      Potential self-helpers (ISH)
  (–) Lacks power for action
      Knowledge not always totally accurate

Contrasexual Ego States (Jung, 1961)
  (+) Balanced personality
      Latent potentials
      Gatekeeper function (?)
  (–) Role diffusion

Shadow (Jung, 1961)
  (+) Creative impulse may originate here
  (–) Potential for evil

False Self, Narcissistic Image
  (+) Protects against infantile helplessness
      Comfort, companionship
  (–) Prevents growth and actualization

persecutors and their look-alikes. Brutal crimes of violence are often their handiwork (Beahrs, 1982b, Appendix II), and confinement in a prison or state hospital is often necessary for the protection of society. For meaningful change to occur, this patient must let go of his need to redress old grievances, but this forgiveness flouts his basic human need for fairness, apparently at his own expense. For the "avenger" ego state, making the ultimate moral choice — seeking vengeance or granting forgiveness (see the Epilogue) — may feel like a non-negotiable demand for suicide.

Many therapeutic dilemmas follow from conflicted multiple consciousness. When parts are in conflict, what feels good to one may feel like a betrayal to another, stirring up insurmountable resistance. When the stakes are high the therapist must set priorities. *Protection must always be the number one priority* when rapport and safety conflict, since nobody can help anyone either dead or sentenced to life imprisonment. Other dilemmas are addressed in *Unity and Multiplicity* (Beahrs, 1982b): whether to treat a person as a unity or a multiple; validation vs. protection; fusion vs. peaceful coexistence; moral choice; and minimizing regressive dependency. Each case must be dealt with in its own unique manner.

If we view the human mind like a symphony orchestra, it is easy to imagine the many ways that the orchestra can go wrong in comparably analogous terms. The string and wind sections could be glaring at each other from within fortified trenches, shelling and lobbing grenades at one another, or they can carry out a campaign of deception and sabotage. A saboteur might set fire to the conductor's coattails while in concert, not unlike Bach and Torbet's (1983) "Inner Enemy." Or the conductor might pass out over the podium with a bottle of whiskey while the members exuberantly party it up. Two or more section leaders might vie for the conductor's baton, or members at large might play "pass it around" with the baton. In dealing with a complex psychotherapy case, I often find it useful to delineate how the patient's inner orchestra is organized, and then how this is going wrong.

Where it is not obvious from the patient's presenting history, this type of information often can be elicited from "internal self-helpers" (ISH) (Allison, 1974), the most significant contribution to the recent practice of ego state therapy. Resembling hidden observers in normal hypnosis, they appear to be sectors of personality with relatively few defining traits of their own, but with a broad factual knowledge of the patient's issues that transcends his usual internal boundaries between ego states. Lacking power for independent action, they function in some ways like "spirit guides" that can alert a therapist to dynamics otherwise missed and suggest hazards to be avoided as well as approaches that might prove fruitful.

With comprehensive knowledge achieved at the expense of power for action, these internal self-helpers or hidden observers may in some ways concretize that yet unknown organizing force that gives a normal person his sense of unity in the face of the multiple co-conscious ego states we all possess. It deserves the most vigorous research effort to define its parameters.

With the incongruities, complexities, and therapeutic binds that multiple consciousness presents us, a therapist needs simple working principles for a sense of stability. Following the lead of Berne (1972), transactional analysts neatly summarize the essence of good psychotherapy as the "three P's": permission, protection, and potency. The *permission* is to simply be, and includes all the basic attributes of an individual's self-identity including those aspects or parts that often appear persecutory. *Protection* makes it safe to simply be and must be granted to all parties concerned, internal and external. When the first two P's appear to conflict, protection comes first for reasons already discussed. *Potency* is the ability to enforce the protection, making the permissions safe. I personally find the three P's to be as good as any simple working principle, but believe that a fourth is required: *priorities*. When different levels conflict, and what works for one is negative to another, we need to decide which takes precedence. This often comes down to personal and professional values. In psychiatric practice, however, protection must always remain number one.

It is also useful to break down the first "P" into three permissions:

1) *permission to be*, which includes not only basic existence but those aspects we usually consider basic to our identity—permission to be who we are, the sex we are, to change and grow, to be childlike, to be important, to be a separate person, etc. It is not always easy to define what this "who we are" actually is, but for disorders that usually result from threat to survival, existential permission is critical;

2) *permission to let things happen*, the trusting spontaneity required for healthy living, exemplified especially by the functions of sleep and sex; and

3) *permission to be in charge*, which respects the executive authority given
to our voluntary free will or the "I," most critical for time structure and directing life plans.

The distinction between voluntary and involuntary action is not
understood biologically, and co-consciousness shows their boundary
to be blurred and relative to perspective. Yet most healthy living
depends on a functional coordination between these levels, and on what
level an action is believed to occur may determine a person's disposi-
tion in a court of law. Optimally, the two reinforce one another. Paradoxically, knowing that we are in charge makes it feel safer to let
things happen, and to be able to let things happen puts us more truly
in charge.

A second case history follows illustrating the discussion of polar opposites and uncertainty.

CASE 2. THE MULTIPLE NONMULTIPLE

Sarah was a 35-year-old woman admitted to a locked psychiatric
ward following a violent suicide attempt. Mental status examination
revealed clear criteria for major depression, but with less vegetative
signs and more internal anger than in the classic case. History revealed
the presence of prolonged periods of elevated mood that probably met
criteria for manic episodes, thus warranting a diagnosis of bipolar affective disorder. However, changes between one affective extreme and
the other were often sudden, responsive to environmental events, and
accompanied by only partial recall. Sarah demonstrated physical intolerance to most psychotropic medications including lithium, antipsychotics, and antidepressants. Thus, I also entertained the possibility
of an atypical dissociative disorder similar to Mrs. R, if not frank multiple personality. Attempts to address and mediate alternate ego states
were bitterly fought off by the patient, however, who remained regressed and self-destructive, often cutting herself in flagrant violation
of clear no-suicide contracts. The stormy initial course even included voluntarily submitting to involuntary commitment on one occa-
sion for the sake of protection.

A point was reached when I chose not to take any further external
measures toward her protection such as involuntary commitment, even
when her alarm signals were extreme. Her life was in her hands, she

was now told; I could only trust her and hope for the best. This risk, with its associated respect for her boundaries, proved a turning point. Interestingly, the patient unwittingly sabotaged a formerly excellent insurance coverage and now could afford only one session per month. It was at this point that treatment became productive and moved forward. I chose to deal with her only as a unified whole person, focusing on developmental issues of the narcissistic and borderline personality as described by Masterson (1981).

The focal intervention was simply repeated guarantees of her safety from any real or symbolic violation by myself, accompanied by strong assertion of my own boundaries. The developmental issues dealt with included trust/mistrust, dependency/autonomy, separation/abandonment, seduction/violation, safety, and the classic narcissistic tension between ideal self-image and true self so thoroughly described by Lowen (1983), Miller (1979), and many others.

Only late in the course of treatment was a diagnosis of multiple personality clear and unambiguous. The patient described a history of many clear and distinct alternate personalities, each of whom had carried different names, personality styles, social associations, and widely divergent but well-developed handwriting styles; these had antedated treatment by several decades. In actual practice, however, I did not once diverge from a unified whole-person frame of reference or make any attempt to purposefully elicit part-selves, and only rarely asked their opinion from the point of view of a hidden observer as mediator. When alternate personalities presented spontaneously, I took them seriously, but responded to them as important aspects or facets of personality, never losing track of other elements hidden at the moment.

While many narcissistic vulnerabilities remained, Sarah was able to terminate treatment with a satisfactory creative adjustment achieved by entry into an unusual lifestyle that appeared to be an adequate arrangement among her many disparate and often conflicting needs, wishes, and desires.

POLAR OPPOSITES AND THE UNCERTAINTY PRINCIPLE

Whether to diagnose and treat Sarah as a whole person or as a multiple illustrates the problem of polar opposites. On the one hand, we are each multiple as evidenced by the impressive data on co-consciousness described earlier. Yet, it is equally true that we are each a whole person, even Sarah — one body, one brain, and the need for a unified sense of identity and direction. Leonard, like many multiple personalities, could not get well until his multiplicity was addressed, the component parts identified, and conflicts mediated. For Sarah, however, treatment as a whole person was essential, even though she was much more clearly a true multiple personality.

I know no way to predict in advance which position in a dichotomy like this will be needed. One rigidly obsessive compulsive character, for example, may welcome permission to "loosen up" and become more flexible, as encouraged by the avant-garde treatments of the 1960s. Another patient, identical in basic psychiatric structure, might perceive any permission to loosen up as a threat to his basic integrity. For the second otherwise identical individual, he would be better *confronted* with his "looseness," thereby being encouraged to become even more deeply rooted in his basic integrity. Only from this sense of greater safety, could he then experiment with new ways of relating — loosening up being a desired side effect. We must look at both sides of the structure/flexibility dichotomy, recognizing that one is best achieved not at the expense of the latter, but often as a condition for the latter. They coexist, side by side, just like the hypnosis and nonhypnosis discussed earlier.

Comparable dichotomies abound and pervade all human living; these are summarized in Figure 5.2, the polarities and paradoxes list. Representative of a wide range of human experience, this list is still by no means complete. I will briefly discuss several different ways in which polar concepts are contrasted with or distinguished from their opposites. The manner in which one concept is contrasted with its converse varies and is not always well understood, and may be different depending upon the level or perspective from which it is viewed. For example, matter and antimatter are often considered true opposites, neutralizing one another with a violent annihilation when brought into contact. However, they could be seen as similar if viewed from another perspective, being "organized energy" or energy with mass. Hence, matter/antimatter as a collective would be one pole of another dichotomy, contrasted with pure or massless energy.

At the psychological level, similar distinctions can be made between depression and mania, being considered opposite extremes of mood.

Figure 5.2. Polarities and paradoxes

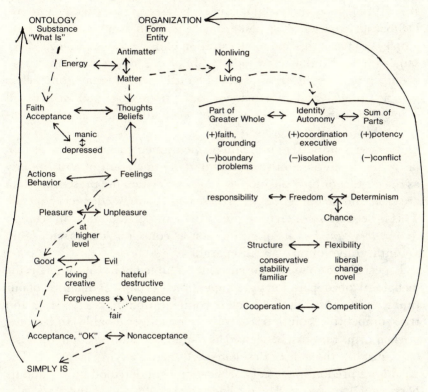

However, both can be considered manifestations of antifaith, or failure to accept and endorse the basic being of self and others. From this perspective, depression/mania would together comprise one pole of another dichotomy, its opposite being a state of faith or basic healthy well-being.

The unity/multiplicity contrast is different in that it is never one *or* the other. A person is simultaneously unified, comprising many parts, and a part of a greater whole; which point of view to take must remain a matter of utility, as illustrated by the cases of Leonard and Sarah (p. 103 and p. 108). Equality vs. uniqueness is a highly politicized variant of this second type of dichotomizing, very evident in today's society.

More subtle intricacies are found in the somewhat parallel motivational dichotomies of pleasure/pain, good/evil, and acceptance/nonacceptance (see Chapter 3). Getting much of their motivating force from an indelible association with pleasure and pain (Spinoza, 1677/1951), good and evil nonetheless transcend the latter dichotomy. Deliberate experience of "pain" may be good in some settings, for example, such as in disciplined frustration of undesirable or illegal drive satisfactions. Similarly, while we abhor the destructive and cruel events in human history that are obviously evil, we may nonetheless give acceptance and endorsement to the nature of mankind with all of its foibles, and the process of cultural evolution that has always constituted human history.

The two compulsive individuals mentioned earlier in this section illustrate the impossibility of defining any one point of a dichotomy as the correct or only position to take, even when the presenting data are clear and unambiguous as in these two otherwise identical patients. This is because so often each pole can be understood only in relation to and *coexistent with* its opposite, just as conscious/unconscious and voluntary/involuntary are inseparable.

Especially germane to our currently troubled political climate is the dichotomy of cooperation vs. competition, perhaps *the* dilemma of our times, as the possibility of nuclear conflagration makes the tried and true competitive "solutions" of warfare no longer tenable. In fact, the nuclear arms race can be viewed as a simple escalating circular causal loop, just like the case of Problematic Punctuation in Chapter 1. The need for a predominance of cooperation is understood by all, and its possibility demonstrated by the effectiveness of many complex societies that have functioned for extended periods of time. But no government has yet forgotten the lesson of Munich, when Neville Chamberlain's attempts to "cooperate" with Hitler not only failed to make the world safe, but guaranteed the worst conflagration of human history. To emphasize one pole at the expense of its opposite is to invite catastrophe. This is the situation with which all world leaders are grappling today. Comparable dilemmas pervade all smaller social contexts such as the workplace and marriage and family, the substrate of much of psychotherapy.

Multilevel functioning along so many different continua introduces the most fundamental root of the uncertainty principle. In fact, it is coexistence of the irreconcilable wave and particle aspects of pure energy that underlies the uncertainty principle in quantum physics. The more precisely we describe a system as a wave, for example, the more uncertainty is introduced in the particle aspect, and vice versa. Precision in the entire system would require precise formulation of *both*, precluded by the inherent duality in a way that is clearly demonstrable empirically but may never be fully understood. The presence of so many comparable dichotomies in human living makes the uncertainty principle even more pervasive and less amenable to quantification.

The foremost implication of uncertainty is that multiple consciousness is virtually inevitable, circularity being avoided by the hard data on multiple consciousness cited earlier. If having effective power for action requires both precision and reliability that can be achieved only at the expense of scope, we can have the best of both worlds if we split into many parts, roles, and ego states, each of which retains power for action in different specialized areas. Working together has the advantages of differentiation, specialization, or division of labor; that which has consistently favored multicellular organisms and complex societal groups throughout the animal kingdom. While the mind–brain seems to have an inherent capacity for simultaneous overlapping patterns of activity that defy explanation in physical science terms, the positive trade-off is the flexibility and the adaptability for which the human brain is legendary.

This is functional co-consciousness and does not require adherence to any one particular psychodynamic model. Furthest from resolution is why and how we have a *sense* of cohesive selfhood and why the self proper is associated with only a small portion of one's conscious experience, the remainder generally considered outside, beyond, "not-me," or, that misnomer, unconscious. And why is that sense of unified self among our most cherished possessions? What is the organizing force or mental glue that holds us together? Who is the conductor? These questions must await further study.

6

The Orthodox
and the Fringe

OVERVIEW

This chapter addresses the state of the mental health profession as a whole, in terms similar to the conductor-orchestra analogy that I have applied to the human mind. Like the mind, our profession is a complex system with a unifying theme. It is divided into many theoretical belief systems and subsystems whose premises often contradict one another and predicate treatment modalities as different as night and day. The purpose of this chapter is to examine why this subdividing is a necessary process, and how to make that process work for us rather than against us. Instead of pitting one system against another, the desired goal is for the mental health profession to function more as an orchestra, with each modality contributing its own unique voice to a cooperative greater whole, under the organizing leadership of an executive, the conductor.

I will pay especially close attention to examining the tension between the psychiatric orthodoxy and the many cults and fads that operate on the fringe, likening this split to the pathological dissociation that defines a multiple personality. The goal in each case is to foster open information exchange so that we can utilize the best that all the component parts have to offer. In the profession as a whole, we want to preserve the creative innovation that often arises at the fringe in any discipline and for this to be anchored in the protective grounding that only an orthodoxy can provide.

114

Campbell (1981) defines psychiatry as "the medical specialty concerned with the study, diagnosis, treatment, and prevention of behavior disorders" (p. 495). If we leave out the limiting word *medical*, and use *mental* and *behavior* interchangeably, this definition can just as well define the mental health profession as a whole. The word *modality* refers to either "any method or technique of treatment," or more broadly to "any class or group within the therapeutic armamentarium" (Campbell, 1981, p. 391). For this discussion, I will use the word in this broader sense. When I use the word *system* in this context, I am referring primarily to a system of beliefs organized around a common premise, those beliefs that are used either to derive a new modality or to justify one in current use. In actual practice "modality" and "system" are virtually indistinguishable from one another, so I will often use the words interchangeably.

All psychiatric systems and treatment modalities share the four key features cited by Frank (1973) as common to all therapy: 1) a *setting* in which evaluation and treatment is carried out; 2) a trusting *relationship*, which is its interpersonal vehicle; 3) a theoretical *rationale* or belief system; and 4) a *treatment method* presumed to be based on the rationale. The last two factors are the key to understanding why psychiatry cannot be unified into a single theoretical and therapeutic system that is both precise and reliable, yet fully comprehensive. For treatment techniques to be more than haphazard and free of the therapist's whim, they must be based on a rationale that has adequate precision and independent validation. Yet so many complex causal factors, polar opposites, and personality variables countervene that almost any belief or belief system has major exceptions. The more narrowly we specify the beliefs, the more likely it becomes that other factors will render them invalid. They will apply to a fewer number of cases, thus have a smaller scope or domain.

Where they do not apply, another system will be needed, with a different rationale and associated treatment techniques. To cover the whole field many systems will be needed. For every clinical situation it is necessary not only to determine which treatments to employ, but to decide which theoretical system will help us define the patient's problems in the first place. I am proposing that the psychiatrist specifically accept this role in the mental health profession — he becomes the conductor who decides which orchestra section to call forth.

Orthodoxy refers to the characteristic of "conforming to established doctrine," or is "conventional" (*Webster's Dictionary*, 1963); *establishment* is what has gained full recognition as an accepted order of society. I will use the words interchangeably to denote mainstream mental health. Orthodox beliefs are those that would be acceptable, even if not fully endorsed, by the majority of practicing psychiatrists; that which one could confortably espouse at a professional meeting. The *fringe* refers to an individual or "group with marginal or extremist views" not accepted by the mainstream. A *cult* is "a system for the cure of disease based on dogma set forth by its promulgator"; "a system of religious beliefs and ritual"; "its body of adherents." A *fad* is simply a "practice or interest followed for a time with exaggerated zeal" (*Webster's Dictionary*, 1963).

Cults and fads can be further distinguished from modalities in the following ways:

1) They are of questionable scientific validity;
2) they are practiced on the fringe without integration into the scientific community at large
3) polarized viewpoints are often held for or against their value, and have more in common with religious sensitivity than objectivity;
4) they often suffer wide swings in popularity that follow sociocultural trends more than growth of scientific data base; and
5) cults take "always" and "never" positions so that their own limits of relevance are frequently transgressed.

Associated treatment techniques may be used indiscriminately, and at best are ineffectual or at worst harmful.

It is important to note that the definitions of the fringe — cults and fads — contain no reference at all to the quality of their associated beliefs and methods, their truth value, or utility. I refer to these as their "legitimacy." To further clarify what defines a legitimate social group, even if on the fringe, Ken Wilber (1983) lists the following features:

1) It is *transrational*, not prerational. In other words, it does not confuse the regressive cognition of wish fulfillment with expansive thinking;
2) legitimacy is anchored in a tradition, like that provided by the great religions;

3) the authority figure is *phase-specific* to the member's developmental
   needs, like schoolteacher or coach who is an appropriate authority
   only at a particular phase of a person's life;
4) it is "NOT headed by a Perfect Master; and
5) it is not out to save the world."

It is not obvious why some questionable models are readily em-
braced by the scientific establishment while others of equal or greater
scientific validity exist only along the fringe as cults or fads separated
from the mainstream by a barrier of mutual antipathy. Adequate supporting data and compatibility with prevailing assumptions certainly act to promote acceptance of a model into the scientific community at large. It is easy to understand that use of tricyclic medication
to relieve depression is widely accepted and the occult therapies would
be kept at arm's length. Yet other factors must play a role, since what
was once a cult often becomes today's accepted modality, and what
is today's mainstream may just as easily become tomorrow's cult.

Social acceptance may be determined by many factors, only one
of which is scientific validation. Psychoanalysis is a good example. It
had only begun to extend beyond cult status during Freud's lifetime,
but within two decades it had become the dominant force in the psychiatric establishment. At its peak, it was virtually impossible for one
to achieve stature in the psychiatric profession without psychoanalytic credentials. But with the resurgence of biological psychiatry since
the advent of effective psychotropic drugs, psychoanalysis has once
again receded into the background, where it again has assumed some
of the social features of cult status.

Starr (1982) describes a similar evolution in the state of organized
medicine. Functioning more like a cult at the time of the American
Revolution, it has become one of the dominant forces that is shaping
our current social structure. According to Starr, this was neither logical
nor necessary, but an outgrowth of the societal forces that can only
be called historical. And the privileged status of medicine is now
threatened by many other socioeconomic forces: economic competition with hospitals and nonmedical therapists, and increasing intrusion of third parties into such determinants as legal liability, quality
assurance, and cost containment.

Other systems have proven to be enduring over long periods of time,
but have persisted in fringe status without ever getting full social

ratification. A few occult systems such as astrology, shamanism, and "past lives" fit into this group; they have persisted because of their considerable personal appeal to many people, but remain too speculative in nature to produce more tangible validation.

Most troublesome is the difficulty we have in distinguishing unredeemable cultism from the highest creative innovation. Like a cult-prone therapist, scientists also look for easy answers, and Teller (1980) even defines science as the "pursuit of simplicity." A hallmark of genius is to look where no one else looks and find something; and we know well that such monumental advances as Copernican astronomy and natural evolution found acceptance only after surviving a long struggle on the fringe. Whether a new idea will prove to be a major breakthrough or a passing fad cannot be decided from the phenomenology alone—it requires information. This is obtained by the scientific method of observation and testing described in Chapter 7, along with the historical dialectic of dominating argument. But the practicing clinician cannot afford to await a verdict of history that is not yet in on the many models currently active on our profession's fringe.

The bottom line that should guide our judgment in difficult decisions is the therapeutic presumption that favors the accepted data base, the establishment and the orthodoxy. The burden of argument is upon he who whould try the unusual, to demonstrate convincingly that what our psychiatric mainstream has to offer this particular patient is unacceptable and/or inadequate, and that an alternative approach has at least a reasonable chance of better results without major complications. Creative innovation is thereby permitted without sacrifice of basic professional protection.

I will present two cases to illustrate the problems of psychiatric cultism and the difficulty in separating this from creative innovation. The first, illustrating cult dynamics, is a clinical case history of an individual who immersed himself in a cult for a full decade and finally extricated himself, but only at great emotional cost. This case will explore the nature of the cult process and the various roots of cultism, including the cognitive roots of circular argument and the fallacy of confusing regressive with transcendent phenomena. Affective roots include many acceptance/nonacceptance dilemmas, as well as economic factors and social cohesiveness of different factions. Narcissistic roots include a particular type of cult-prone leader who attracts a complementary type of cult-prone follower — both crave easy answers. When splitting within our profession becomes truly dysfunctional, there are also many features reminiscent of post-traumatic dissociation in multiple personalities and victims of post-traumatic stress disorder, which are reviewed at this new social level.

The second case is that of a brilliant practitioner who has neither attempted nor succeeded in establishing a common purpose with the professional mainstream, but who has become expert at one after another unusual or unorthodox system. This case is especially important in illustrating where social aspects of cultism are present alongside the potential for considerable creative innovation. Several areas of psychiatry's domain are examined with regard to where they stand within our profession vis-à-vis the orthodox/fringe dimension. These include hypnosis and multiple personality, which are rapidly moving toward broad acceptance; psychic phenomena, which remain on the fringe; and a group of unexplained biological phenomena that are addressed by a discipline called clinical ecology.

I agree with Starr that many societal factors determine such an area's social status of which legitimacy as I have defined it on p. 000 is only one. I simply urge that we keep an open mind about all the underlying phenomena that a modality attempts to deal with, whether or not they can be explained, and whether or not they fit current paradigms. Two common fallacies need to be avoided: 1) the risk of equating unorthodoxy with invalidity; and 2) equating "not yet explained" with "does not exist." The chapter closes with suggested criteria for employing an unorthodox theoretical rationale and/or associated treatment modality.

CASE 1. THE CULTIST

Kenneth was a young man seen on referral from another psychiatrist for chronic depression, trancelike states, and a general inability to organize and take charge of his direction in life. He had been raised in an upwardly mobile Protestant family whose achievement-oriented values he largely accepted. Under the stress of a difficult academic studies program, he had become frustrated, disillusioned, and quietly desperate. Occasional use of hallucinogenic drugs simply supported the temporary comfort of "tuning out," while he slipped further behind in his own self-advancement. He was ripe for a charismatic guru, and sure enough one proved to be available at just the right time.

A dramatic conversion swept over Kenneth, who now "saw" the emptiness of his entire life with its emphasis on material values, as well as the futility of tuning out on drugs. He "saw" that the guru had the answer: to escape "ordinariness" and achieve a higher consciousness and oneness with the absolute — all that really mattered — required giving up old habits and associations in favor of a disciplined adherence to the newly found Way. With a sense of relief and an exhilarating sense of freedom, he felt everything fitting into place. His life now had meaning, supported by the wise direction provided by the teachings of his guru. At times his elation was accompanied by ecstatic visual hallucinations, which further reinforced the sense of divine origin of his conversion. Furthermore, he felt like he was now among friends as never before, and could see himself as one of an elite few who, through cooperative effort, would save the world from its own self-destructiveness. While his bereaved and now estranged family reported him as looking glazed, as if in a trance, all he himself experienced was a pervasive warm glow.

Why Kenneth became disillusioned with his cult is not entirely clear: perhaps continued pressure from his family who had not yet given up hope; perhaps an inner revulsion toward the shadier practices of cult members, violating his own original reason for joining; perhaps the tedium of never-ending cult discipline; perhaps simple maturation; probably for some or all of these and other reasons. Years before he broke from his cult he tortured himself with doubts. Would he be betraying the only real friends he had ever had? Might he be abandoning the true God after all? Worse yet, would he be hunted down and exterminated by his former comrades for his betrayal? But overruling those concerns, the warm glow had become tiresome and Kenneth craved the sharp edge of ordinary living.

The treatment contract was simple: training in *nonhypnosis*. The patient's spontaneous trances were so dysfunctional that he needed to reexert voluntary control over his own mind and relearn skills from the *non*hypnotic end of the continuum. This included greater awareness of trance states when they spontaneously occurred, using these as signals to reassert voluntary control over his actions and experience. It involved coaching him on the use of a crisp, organized, informative, and directional style of language. Most important, his task was to realistically assess his goals and options. The modest outgrowth of all this was a more healthy acceptance of the value of simple ordinary living. In his own words, it is "more blessed to peel carrots than to seek Nirvana"—a holdover from cultish-type thinking to be sure, but at least an auspicious start in a more healthy direction.

NARCISSISTIC ROOTS: THE CULT PROCESS

Many factors can make a man such as Kenneth vulnerable to cultism. Not the least is the cult's implicit offer of relief from the ongoing stress of autonomous adult living and the many disagreeable aspects of reality itself. If there appears to be an "easy way," it can have significant attractive power to the naive; this is the drawing card of the cult. Unresolved childhood dependency needs also make one vulnerable to such groups. If the individual has already warded off the pain of a traumatic childhood with a defensive false self, he is further vulnerable. Any "easy way" whose world view fits that of the false self will have the support of his neurotic defense mechanisms.

Other vulnerabilities are more phase-specific. First, the hard knocks of reality may deflate the narcissistic grandiosity of an earlier developmental stage. Although a healthy process, this is still extremely painful to the individual involved, who may be especially receptive at this time to any position that restores a sense of being special. Second, and just as important, is entry into Piaget's cognitive stage of formal operations (Flavell, 1963). For the first time in his life, a person is now able to see objective reality as just a special case of what is possible. Reality no longer seems so pretty when compared to the greener pastures of the imagination, and it is certainly not fair. At the bottom line, the cult convert has a profound experience that things can be different. An alternative reality without the usual stresses and strains is the cult's siren song.

Once the cult-prone individual enters his cult something snaps. It seems that reality has truly changed to fit his ideal images. The sense of relief is exhilarating, and has the ineffable quality of a mystical experience (James, 1902/1961), or what Freud (1930/1961) referred to as *oceanic feeling*, which I will use interchangeably with *cult affect*. This feeling has many of the same qualities of traumatic affect described earlier, not only in being hard to describe, but also in being accompanied by many hypnotic experiences. But instead of being aversive, it is maximally attractive. Cult affect is therefore like a mirror image of traumatic affect, in which helplessness is replaced by an emotional sense of omnipotence.

To others it looks like the new convert is in a hypnotic trance. The warm glow, the trancelike appearance, visual hallucinations, and the dependence on suggestions from a dominant other all fit that description. This is compatible with Galanter's (1982) observation that atypical dissociative disorder is a frequent manifestation of the cult process, since dissociative disorders appear to be disorders of spontaneous hypnosis, and hypnosis itself involves dissociation. There can be no doubt that at the time of entry into the cult, the patient had "split." Values as firmly based as those by which he had been raised could hardly have disappeared. But they were certainly not evident — they had gone underground.

The cult process therefore shares two essential features with traumatic dissociation: 1) it is driven and fueled by a powerful affect that is hard to describe in terms of ordinary human feelings; and 2) it is associated with the volitional, perceptual, and cognitive alterations that define what we call hypnotic. Hence, it can be illustrated by a similar type of schematic diagram to that used in the last chapter (Fig. 5.1, p. 100). But the question is, how can that occur, even in the absence of gross abuse or threat to survival, and when the associated feelings are most pleasant?

The cult process is illustrated in Figure 6.1. As in the case of intrapsychic trauma, a sector of personality is split off from the greater body of self that maintains contact with reality. All that differs is the nature of the affect that drives the process. After gross trauma, reality had become so aversive that normal coping required it to be pushed aside. With cult formation it is the mirror inverse. Reality may or may not be so bad, but the cult reality is so attractive that the differential is the same. Whether by a push or a pull, reality is avoided. The many small arrows again refer to the forces that push away the true reality-oriented self in order to preserve the illusionary cult reality. And the few larger arrows refer to intrusion of this greater self into the complacency of the cult self. The tradeoff is also the same — relative comfort is bought at the sacrifice of true selfhood and at the price of perpetuating the split.

Figure 6.1. The cult process

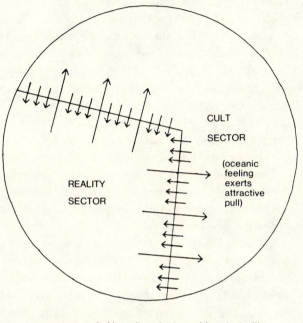

energy expended by cult sector to avoid contact with
potentially corrective outside reality and the
reality-oriented self

intrusions of reality-oriented self into the
complacency of the cult sector

As Galanter (1982) had noted for cults in general, Kenneth had
found a consensual belief system, social cohesiveness, the security of
group norms oriented around a common purpose, and a charismatic
leader to whom he could delegate responsibility for direction in his
own life. He had found an easy answer. From the point of view of
the cult itself, its very isolation allowed it to be a laboratory in which
it could carry out its mission relatively free of societal interference.

Although the mutual boundary assertion between the cult and
society at large feels so protective, it prevents information exchange.
For all practical purposes, the cult is walled off from contact with outside information, and the benefits of society are therefore denied. Cult
beliefs are therefore inadequately tested and may lead to problematic

actions that even our profession's current knowledge would render untenable. In addition, the very real issues of society as a whole simply are not addressed. Regressive dependency is also a frequent concomitant, an almost essential element in cult maintenance.

The bottom line is that the cultist has chosen an *image* of self and reality that is idealized, *not real* — it has very little connection with the macrocosm of human society. Whether trauma and overwhelming stress render the greater reality untenable or whether an illusory easy answer appears, a patient with high hypnotizability may split, essentially using "trance as a coping mechanism" (Frankel, 1976). Conflicted areas are put aside behind a dissociative barrier, resulting in a Faustian tradeoff: The conflict-free sector of personality is now able to grow, develop, and function without interference from the conflict itself, but this is achieved at great cost; the problem is never addressed and resolved, and thereby persists.

As we have seen in Chapter 5, the phenomena of ideal self-image versus real self links the concepts of post-traumatic stress disorder, pathological narcissism, and life scripts. Perhaps it is a common thread across the gamut of all mental disorders with primarily psychological origin. An ideal image is not pathological per se; it is only when it is confused with the true self at the very deepest level of thinking that a severe personality disorder or equivalent may result.

In interpersonal terms, there is a unique type of symbiotic interaction between a cult-prone therapist and a cult-prone patient such as Kenneth. The former is often a grandiose and rebellious individual with an immense sense of insecurity and dissatisfaction, who feels estranged from others and seeks a simple solution that both relieves his dysphoria and grandiosity. The latter is a tormented individual who for many reasons may require an external authority to feel all right, and who, like his potential guru, also craves easy answers. It is as if the two are made for one another, and when they get together they are apt to bask in their narcissistic glow, ignoring all data and all models that would challenge their system.

This section has described what I call the narcissistic roots of cultism, the tension between the ideal and the real that Lowen (1983) considers the essence of narcissism. Other factors contribute to cultism — cognitive, social, cultural, and economic — some of which are described in the next section.

COGNITIVE ROOTS OF CULTISM

Cognitive roots of cultism are twofold, circularity and the Pre/Trans Fallacy (Wilber, 1983). Circular thinking is using a premise to derive some conclusion that is then used to derive the original premise, and so on, ignoring objective data that could be corrective. Circularity infiltrates human thinking at almost all levels, from reverberating circuits in the brain to complex theoretical systems, and probably plays an important role in helping us maintain stable organized thinking patterns in the face of awesome perceptual complexity (Hebb, 1949).

Any adequate scientific theory needs to be internally consistent, which means that different parts of the theory can be logically deduced from others. This is a type of circularity. But scientific consistency is circularity grounded in objective data. This is what gives the theory its legitimacy. Circularity is a problem only when potentially corrective information is excluded.

The antithesis to circular thinking is not logic, since there is a self-justifying and often irrefutable logic to the circular system. The antidote is corrective information. In the scientific realm, this comes in the form of carefully structured systematic observation and is confirmed by the controlled experiment and statistical validation. When an element in a circular system is clearly disproven, it may become necessary to discard or drastically rework the entire system. Where this type of validation is not possible because the data cannot be measured or tested, freedom of debate offers another antithesis by ensuring that contradictory viewpoints will be given equal voice. This is the basis of the adversary system of Anglo-American law. It is also the mechanism that forces children to give up primitive magical thinking in favor of concrete logic (Flavell, 1963).

When circular reasoning becomes problematic, this corrective information is forcefully excluded. As we saw with Kenneth, he had isolated himself from the entire fund of human knowledge by his cult's boundary formation, supported by the emotional pull of oceanic feeling.

Ken Wilber (1983) describes another cognitive root of cultism, which he calls the Pre/Trans Fallacy. He maintains that the primitive magical thinking of the toddler stage is easily confused with the "unitary" stage (Koplowitz, 1984), a more advanced level of cognitive development. Neither are bound to concrete or formal logic, and both may be associated with attractive feelings. But one is "below," the other "beyond." To confuse these two, as the cultist often does, is to take the risk of rationalizing regressive dependency as if it were a new advance in the progress of human knowledge.

In understanding the logic of cults, there is probably no better example than astrology. An ancient and enduring belief system from which many take comfort and seek direction in life even today, it has proven as difficult to disprove as it has been to support. Neither the sciences of astronomy nor astrophysics have found any objective support for astrological beliefs, which remain speculative and isolated from scientific testing. Nonetheless, many individuals with an otherwise adequate intellectual curiosity and healthy scientific skepticism continue to subscribe to these beliefs.

It is understandable how this incongruity occurs in view of the comprehensive but nonspecific nature of astrological charts or horoscopes, and the multiplicity inherent in human consciousness. A quality horoscope, for example, is not sufficiently specific to be proven or disproven, but denotes a relative preponderance of certain traits and characteristics, all of which all human beings possess to some degree. If it does not fit the person's conscious self-image, it might at least validate some hidden potentials. The chart then might act as a therapeutic double bind, as follows: If the chart fits, the subject experiences it as a validation, e.g., "I'm a Taurus, and I'm OK — that's just the way I am." If it does *not* fit, his attention will be called to latent abilities that he had not formally been aware of but that are there, and may develop these in a new direction. In either case, the horoscope would have a positive effect and support itself.

Using astrology in daily living is not necessarily positive, however. There are disturbed marriages in which one party has used the other's astrological chart as a bludgeon with which to hammer the spouse, eventually leading to dissolution of the marriage. Whether these marriages would have dissolved anyway or whether it is for the best is unclear; it is equally possible that without the convenient rationalizations, the parties might have sought and discovered more mature solutions to their conflict and moved ahead to greater intimacy.

Circular reasoning is not unique to astrology or cults. It encompasses thinking at its highest levels. The commonly quoted phrase, "the devil can cite Scripture for his purpose," points toward the circularity in Christian ethics. Psychoanalysis is also well known for its ability to explain almost any psychological event *ex post facto* whatever the actual data. This applies almost as much to other psychodynamic theories and is probably essential for the integrity and stability of our lives.

There are also social roots of cultism, some of which have already been discussed, including the factors that lead a cult to isolate itself from society and forcefully exclude the information it could contribute. Aspects of the establishment itself that promote cultism are more subtle and pervasive, and deserve close scrutiny. These issues will be discussed following another case presentation, that of a clinical practitioner, in which elements of cultism and creativity are most difficult to tease apart.

CASE 2. THE PROPHET

Dr. M is a 60-year-old physician trained at prestigious academic centers, with subsequent psychiatric training having a psychoanalytic bias, in keeping with the tradition of his era. Initially fascinated by the intellectuality of analytic formulations, he had become disillusioned with his own personal analysis by what seemed to him to be a game without end (see the case Analysis Interminable, p. 76, for a parallel discussion of that phenomenon). He terminated psychoanalytic training mid-stream with a desire to chart his own course. He was first attracted by, then immersed in, several of the body therapies of the 1960s, becoming a widely sought expert in the Gestalt techniques of Perls (1969). He felt that these could break through the empty intellectualizing of psychoanalytic psychiatry and get to the nitty-gritty of life: real feelings and their avoidance.

At first treated with cautious respect by his peers, Dr. M was later kept at arm's length by the professional community for "suspect judgment." He also often contemptuously referred to the members of this establishment as "conventional." Which one preceded the other is not clear, but in any case, the boundary between his teachings and those of the professional establishment became increasingly rigid.

As Dr. M's work became more and more walled off from the scientific community, his clientele changed from young *avant garde* professionals to emotionally disabled patients who were in search of an easy answer. He sounded more and more like a religious teacher, preaching "the true way of life" — a way quite positive on the whole, yet increasingly doctrinaire. He devoted more and more of his energy to a group of severely disturbed patients who he felt could not be helped by establishment psychiatry, and conveyed an attitude toward this clientele that others saw as an attempt to rescue them from themselves. His situation became untenable when many of his new charges often not only failed to appreciate his help, but turned against him. Instead of getting well, the patients sometimes regressed before his eyes with destructive acting out against themselves and others. An alarmed citizenry finally forced Dr. M out of the area, at which time he moved to another community. Many loyal followers moved with him. A cult was in the making.

Fortunately for Dr. M and his work, he recognized the risk of meeting his own needs only through supporting dependent others. Whether or not he appreciated the pathogenic effect of boundary confusion (see Chapter 4), he recognized a need to take care of himself. He joined an accepted if somewhat authoritarian religious sect, achieving a base of social support that has proven satisfactory. He subsequently withdrew from psychosocial psychiatry altogether to become an authority in psychobiology. It is not the psychobiology of mainstream psychiatry, however, but the nutritional approaches and clinical ecology that still function on the fringe. His work is positive, independent, and highly creative, but almost entirely disconnected from the mental health profession as a whole. Not surprisingly, he attracts primarily a clientele with similar biases.

CULTISM VS. CREATIVITY

Several features of cultism are present in the work of Dr. M: 1) for whatever reason, a persisting dissatisfaction with the traditional, accepted data base; 2) latching onto new belief systems as if absolute, both his own and others, excluding the potentially corrective information of our entire profession's collective research; and 3) consensual belief systems shared with an intimate coterie of significant others. His role as guru, rather than follower, is probably a normal outgrowth of maturation and his considerable intellectual prowess. The disadvantage was described already for cults and circular reasoning: Exclusion of corrective information prevents full growth. A system grows, develops, and flourishes, but at the cost of not going past cult status.

Noticeably missing from this discussion so far is any evaluation of the specific content of Dr. M's work. One cannot write it off as necessarily invalid or even unhealthy until taking a closer look at the nature of his beliefs and practices. As Kuhn (1962/1970) has argued, a new scientific paradigm is born of a period of increasing dissatisfaction with the status quo, based on either its factual inadequacies or emotional vulnerabilities of the individuals involved. More often both factors are present, and it is very difficult in actual practice to separate one from the other. Rothstein (1980) argues that all new paradigms follow a sequence of development virtually indistinguishable from the previous description of cultism. History shows that many a creative genius has been dissatisfied with his profession, willfully worked on the fringe with an isolated coterie of followers, and rejected the community at large. And the establishment's initial resistance to such new paradigms as Copernican astronomy, quantum mechanics, and psychoanalysis all show that the pushing aside of discordant beliefs is a two-way street.

The central element in the cult/creativity problem is what to do with *unexplained data* — observable phenomena difficult to understand in terms of the tried and true, and practical problems that elude current technology. Many such phenomena pervade the psychological level; consciousness itself, as well as hypnosis, intrapsychic conflict, multiple personality, and psychic phenomena. None are well understood, and they are professionally accepted to varying degrees. Hypnosis is rapidly moving into the mainstream to the benefit of all concerned. Study of multiple personality is at an earlier stage of a similar process. In each case the move toward acceptance can be credited to their investigators' efforts to follow establishment research guidelines. Psychic phenomena remain on the fringe, due to their intangible quality and the speculative nature of their associated beliefs.

There are similar unexplained phenomena at the biological level in medicine and psychiatry. Among these are the environmental sensitivities studied by clinical ecology, Dr. M's current discipline, isolated from the medical establishment by a wall of mutual antipathy that I cannot understand. With psychobiology at the forefront of our profession, I cannot explain why these phenomena are ignored by mainstream psychiatry and treated as if they do not even exist. I will use the schism between clinical ecology and the mainstream as a springboard for understanding those factors within the establishment itself that promote cultism.

To understand the current status and controversy surrounding clinical ecology, it is best to keep in mind two basic points in addition to its fringe status. First, it embraces a large and nearly comprehensive collection of psychophysiological phenomena that are so far not explained, and apparently not explainable in terms of current medical knowledge. Second, there is a relatively small but still substantial group of practitioners who have a common belief about how these phenomena are best manipulated for therapeutic ends. It is this group of approaches that collectively defines the discipline of clinical ecology. It is most critical to distinguish these two features, that particular beliefs and methods are not to be equated with the phenomena themselves. Beliefs and methods are appropriately subject to acceptance or rejection, but the phenomena simply are, waiting for whatever understanding and utilization lie in the future. The phenomena are as follows:

Numerous individuals seem to be overly sensitive to normally low and nontoxic doses of environmental substances: chemical pollutants, foods, pollens, and related plant dusts. The untoward reactions differ widely among different individuals. Occasionally they follow known patterns of clinical allergy, such as atopic dermatitis, but more often their etiology remains obscure. Symptoms associated with offending agents may include malaise, euphoria, dysphoria of a variety of types, depersonalization reactions, exaggeration of preexisting neurotic traits, and even transient psychosis. Physical symptoms include skin eruptions, respiratory distress, abdominal pain, cramping and bloating, joint aches, tension headaches, and a variety of other musculoskeletal complaints. People "adapt" when frequently exposed to agents that they are sensitive to, and may even crave offending foods in a manner much like an addiction (Randolph, 1956). After a sufficient time has passed since prior exposure, however, they will prove more sensitive then ever. These are the basic phenomena behind clinical ecology: neither true nor false, good nor bad, right nor wrong; simply facts, waiting for some explanation.

Clinical ecologists believe that people exposed to these offending agents over an extended time frequently develop a variety of chronic illnesses, as listed by Bell (1982): "nephrotic syndrome, poststreptococcol nephritis, cardiac arrhythmias, thrombophlebitis, and vasculitis . . . primary hypothydroidism . . . rheumatoid arthritis, migraine headache, and ulcerative colitis" (p. 29). Chronic mental illness is also felt to be a frequent correlate. These are all severe, chronic, and disabling illnesses that have not been adequately explained to date by the medical profession, and even less well treated. They encompass those conditions frequently termed *psychosomatic*, as well as the gamut of rheumatic or autoimmune diseases. When placed in a clean environment free from substances to which they are sensitive, a certain number of these patients show a partial to complete recovery from their illness, over and beyond what is expected from current medical knowledge.

An elaborate clinical program of systematic testing and disciplined avoidance of offending agents has been developed, constituting the current practice of clinical ecology. Reports of therapeutic benefit are manifold; many are presented in a therapeutic compendium edited by Dickey (1976), and the rationale is concisely reviewed by Bell (1982). Without arguing the pros and cons of clinical ecology, I will review those factors that maintain the barrier between this intriguing collection of phenomena and the medical community as a whole, in my opinion to the detriment of both.

Bell (1982) believes that the rejection of clinical ecology by the medical establishment is due to the following factors: 1) lack of rigorous documentation of the basic assumptions; 2) the anecdotal nature of the findings; and 3) the interdisciplinary nature of the work that renders it essentially beyond the scope of any one particular medical specialty — i.e., it "lacks a single traditional field which could accommodate it and test its basic concepts" (p. 24). The prevalence of neuropsychiatric symptomatology pushes it outside the domain of allergy, while toxicologists will not deal with the phenomena because of the subtoxic doses of the agents involved, and idiosyncratic reactions to even healthy foodstuffs are the very substrate of the work. Grieco (1982) simply notes that medical allergists do not share the views of the clinical ecologist.

Brodsky (1983) further criticizes the field because of its social consequences, likening it to a "medical subculture" or cult. He notes that the clientele of clinical ecology often become obsessed with sensitivity to the point that they will avoid virtually anything and everything conceivable, a phobic life position that leads to progressive withdrawal from society.

First (1980) is harshly critical of the establishment, claiming that many selfish factors lead it to reject valid clinical data and techniques that would help many people: 1) willful subversion of communication, such as refusal to include the *Journal of Orthomolecular Psychiatry* in the *Index Medicus*; 2) matters of pride; 3) respect for the authority of his peers; and 4) simple economics. She argues further that orthomolecular psychiatry and its associate, clinical ecology, are paradigms that will necessarily replace the current paradigm of specific etiology.

A more objective evaluation was attempted by Pearson, Rix, and Bentley (1983). They evaluated 23 patients with a variety of symptoms that they attributed to food allergy, the classic complaint of clientele of the clinical ecologist. They were blindly evaluated by a psychiatrist and an allergist, as well as put on an elimination diet devoid of foods to which they reported sensitivity. Only four of the 23 manifested true allergy, and 18 of the other 19 patients met criteria for a significant mental disorder; there was no overlap between the two groups. *All* of the patients reported clinical improvement when placed on an elimination diet, and all reported a worsening when taking the offending agents. However, they were consistently *not* able to identify offending foods on double blind provocation testing. In addition, the investigators noted that these patients 1) had objective evidence of psychiatric disorder, 2) were reluctant to view their problems in psychological terms, and 3) had been exposed to outside information on food allergies that might have served as the content of suggestion. They advised great caution in attributing emotional symptoms to food allergy.

These data can be interpreted in different ways. The most narrow scientific view would be to conclude that the phenomena do not even exist, but are a misinterpretation of other phenomena. Another possibility is that the testing procedure was inadequate — for example, inadequate test doses or interference by the other agents used as a vehicle for the testing. A more intriguing perspective is that the food sensitivities may be significant, but only in combination with other somatic and/or psychological factors, all of which must be present for symptom formation, but most of which were excluded by the experimental design. If complex biopsychosocial interactions are needed to explain certain phenomena, then isolated testing of controlled variables would be expected to yield negative results (Hoffer, 1974). Alternate research strategies would be needed.

The greatest caution is needed not to confuse a negative or equivocal study with "does not exist." Other bizarre psychosomatic phenomena have been documented in multiple personality and felt to be state dependent (Braun, 1984). Even if the phenomena of clinical ecology prove to be little more than a biological face-saver, the magnitude of this phenomenon would still merit close scrutiny. Whatever the future historical verdict on systems like clinical ecology will be, the phenomena remain and demand careful study. So far, this venture has been undertaken only by investigators like Dr. M, who have been willing to remain on the fringe and to be judged as cultists by the rest of us.

In summary, it is human nature for there always to be an orthodoxy and a fringe. The orthodoxy provides stability and protective grounding, while the fringe encourages creative innovation. There is also much splitting within each of these domains. The fringe then develops coexisting "alternative orthodoxies" like clinical ecology that have their own fringe, and so on. The advantages of this splitting process are specialized division of labor, and the freedom each sector has from outside interference. However, the price is paid in internal conflict and blocked information flow. This cost may be minimized by keeping an open mind to unexplained data, and to utilizing unorthodox modalities in a cautious manner that increases their potential benefit and minimizes their risk.

CRITERIA FOR USE OF AN UNORTHODOX MODALITY

To maximize our profession's effectiveness regardless of our professional bias we will do better to make room for a wide variety of alternative treatment strategies that have proven helpful to some patients, even if only infrequently or in unusual circumstances. Yet to transgress beyond the limits of our own educational background would be to risk the type of unredeemed cultism that was so devastating to Kenneth, and to so many troubled youngsters like him. For this reason,

I believe that the burden of proof should always be upon the one trying to employ an unusual or unorthodox system, to demonstrate with clear, cogent, and convincing evidence that the clinical problem in question is atypical, not fitting the traditional model; and that the patient has received an adequate trial of conventional treatment without adequate benefit. Only at this point, more specific signs are then sought that might point toward a specific unusual modality.

Vague allergies, signs of deficiency, and even a "sick look" in the presence of normal medical findings might point toward an ecological or orthomolecular approach. Repetitive maladaptive behavior eluding psychoanalytic, transactional, or behavioral approaches might point toward some occult psychotherapy. If a patient believes in and wants a particular approach, this also should be a relative indication, unless the desired approach is clearly contraindicated, or strong positive evidence supports the more traditional approach.

The overriding principle should be the well-known dictim of *primum non nocere*, or "first do no harm." The burden of argument is upon the one who would try the unusual, to demonstrate convincingly that what the medical and psychiatric mainstream has to offer this particular patient is unacceptable, and that an alternative approach has at least a reasonable chance of better results without major complications. Creative innovation is thereby permitted without sacrificing professional protection.

7

Science and

the Unscientific

OVERVIEW

The scientific method is a complex integrated process that utilizes all levels of thinking from the creative hunch and personal bias to the more rational processes of systematic observation, measurement and testing, and statistical evaluation. The purpose of this chapter is to address the tasks of science, which include the twofold charge of embracing the most information and making maximal effort to test its validity. A major dilemma is determining the place we should give to material that by its very nature cannot be measured or tested, yet crops up so often in the consulting room that to exclude it would be as truly unscientific as to uncritically accept it. This material includes subjective conscious awareness, as well as the paranormal or occult. How to include the untestable aspects of our work into a protective overall scientific superstructure is a major challenge.

Science basically means knowing. Only more recently has the word become indelibly associated with that particular method known as the controlled experiment and its correlate, statistical dominance, both of which contribute to greater certitude that we give those beliefs we call scientific. To assume that these are the only valid sources of scientific data is to embrace a dogma I refer to as *scientism*, whose definition of reality is that which can be measured and tested. According to the scientific dogmatist, for practical purposes anything that cannot be measured and tested does not exist. When a psychiatrist takes this unfortunate position, he has excluded from his armamentarium many of the "soft" intangibles that make human beings human and provide the heart of therapeutic potency.

The subject matter of all scientific inquiry is "reality" or what is. Watzlawick (1976) points out the importance of not confusing our belief systems with the underlying primary reality or "really real," which is beyond description with language. Science can help us develop better and better theories, but these will remain what they are — models only. That there is even a more fundamental reality, such as a forest with trees still visible even when no one is there to view it, must forever remain a matter of faith (Beahrs, 1977a).

Our current deference to the method of controlled experiment ignores the fact that this method is not the primary source of knowing, nor can it ever be. While it is essential for testing the validity of current theories, it is singularly ineffective at gathering the new data that lead to these theories. The psychodynamics of Freud and the cognitive psychology of Piaget were instead based on an alternate method, systematic observation of phenomena that could not be controlled except on a limited basis. Systematic observation is without peer for gathering information or "ruling in." Freud was a master of systematic observation, carefully recording such mental events as dream images, changes in feeling tone, automatic thoughts, parapraxes, and their nonrandom association not only with neurotic symptoms but with many aspects of everyday living. Only later did he develop his psychoanalytic theories (Freud, 1916/1979) to make sense of his data, and only recently have most of these theories been subjected to the test of controlled experiment. Some ideas have passed these tests well, like stages of emotional development, while others have fared less well, like the psychology of women. The task of controlled experiment is to "rule out" clearly false beliefs and establish limits of relevance to others.

These two aspects of the scientific method vary inversely on two important parameters: Systematic observation is high on information yield but very low on validity, while controlled experiment is low on information yield, and high on validity. Adequacy requires both, and the methods reciprocally enhance one another.

A third but nonscientific process should be stated in deference to its dominating role in human thinking — the level of nonrational factors, including the creative hunch. Uncertain in information content and low in validity, it is often the driving force behind the first two processes, and sometimes later proves to have had a more valid basis than originally perceived. Knowing usually starts with the creative hunch, which then directs the focus for systematic observation, leading to hypotheses that can be put to the test of controlled experiment. The creative hunch is considered acceptable when its content is in accord with social convention, though this is clearly not scientific. Freedom of debate is probably the best corrective at this level, assuring us that relevant alternative views will be on the table for scrutiny.

The challenge yet for scientific psychiatry is how to deal with that aspect of reality whose very existence is denied by rigid scientism: that which *cannot* be measured and tested. Two types of nontestable data are especially relevant to psychiatry — subjective awareness and a slippery group of mental phenomena usually referred to as *paranormal* or *occult*. Subjective awareness or consciousness, a traditional philosophical issue reviewed briefly in the overview that opens Chapter 3, is relevant because even though modifying the state of a patient's consciousness is often a psychiatrist's primary task, we cannot know this state in another by any systematic means of measurement, only by his outward communication. The occult phenomena are important for three reasons: 1) we need to keep open to data that challenge current assumptions; 2) dealing with this group of phenomena may help us successfully treat at least a significant minority of troubled patients for whom orthodox methods have failed; and 3) we need to avoid the unnecessary tragedy of mislabeling higher human creativity as psychotic just because it does not fit our preconception of what reality should be. The premises of science are clearly changing, and they must; scientism is meeting its limits.

The relevance of these issues to the practicing clinician can be summarized as follows: Regarding what we do not know we must keep an open mind, and be careful neither to glibly accept nor categorically reject material that jars our basic beliefs. Perhaps the most productive attitude is what Freud (1916/1979) called benevolent skepticism, the attitude recommended that prospective psychoanalytic patients should take. Some patients present with bizarre quasi-delusional thinking, but do not appear seriously deranged; they often seem to be attempting to make sense of some unusual experience that defies explanation. It helps to validate the experience as a phenomenon that is not right or wrong but simply is, distinguishing it from beliefs about the experience, about which appropriate caution is advised.

Other times a disturbed patient might appear to be in a spontaneous hypnotic trance, and simply helping him put the phenomenon under his control will help him change a symptom into a skill (Beahrs, 1982b). Another patient might request that past-life experiences be dealt with and worked through. While the content of these must remain grossly speculative, it is just as illogical to categorically reject as to uncritically accept them. If they do not run afoul of reality at a more tangible level, and if they help a patient solve his conflicts while saving face, there is no reason why we should not honor his request. To accept and utilize a patient's beliefs is a cornerstone of Milton Erickson's contributions (Beahrs, 1982a), and should be increasingly emphasized in the new scientific thinking.

Following is a case that illustrates the fallacy of equating statistical predominance with absolute reality, which leads to a review of that area in psychiatry most limited by this type of scientism, the study of schizophrenia. A second case highlights the importance of data not testable by the controlled experiment, which also reaches toward a scientific method more capable of dealing with data currently beyond our ability to measure and test.

CASE 1. PARANOID EXECUTIVE:
THE UNUSUAL SPECIAL CASE

Mrs. G was an ambitious and hard-driving 36-year-old executive. While she carried an ongoing diagnosis of paranoid schizophrenia, she nonetheless functioned quite competently in a highly demanding executive role, where she showed clear thinking, good judgment, and an ability to act decisively in stressful situations. She had experienced several psychotic episodes with disorganized thinking, and auditory hallucinations telling her that she was no good and should kill herself and that associates and less defined "enemies" were plotting against her. These were all superimposed on a nearly continuous background of suspiciousness and thoughts that people could enter or control her mind, along with a high anxiety level. Except for minimal deterioration of personality, she clearly and unambiguously met all the DSM-

III criteria for paranoid schizophrenia. The continued high level of functioning suggested that we take a closer look.

As in many atypical cases I have described, her response to neuroleptic antipsychotic medication was equivocal. She was unusually sensitive to medication-induced movement disorders, but could be maintained on low doses of haloperidol with noticeable suppression of psychotic behavior. Suspecting an additional component of atypical personality disorder with psychotic manifestations, I also recommended psychotherapy. She proved to be a well motivated and responsive patient, systematically working through a variety of issues such as abandonment, autonomy, and of course, basic trust. The problem was that her clinical status continued virtually as it had for the several years prior to instituting psychiatric treatment.

Following a six-month sabbatical Mrs. G returned. She glowingly claimed to have been free of all psychiatric symptoms for several months. Her thinking was clear and coherent, there was a wider range of objective affect, there were no signs of the ideas of reference that had been so pervasive earlier, and she simply looked better. What had happened? On the advice of a friend, she had seen a fringe practitioner of holistic mental health who had placed her on a regimen of megavitamins. It is sufficient to say that I was impressed.

THE LIMITS OF SCIENTISM

The "unusual special case" just described is one of several illustrating the limits of scientism and its idolatry of the scientific method in the mental health profession. I do not intend to preach a case for megavitamins, and only rarely do I utilize these in my own clinical practice. Rather, Paranoid Executive is cited to reinforce our observation that phenomena occur in a wide variety of areas of human experience that do not fit current explanations. Not all of these are amenable to the controlled experiment and statistical analysis, and some of these may be a bit unnerving. All remain to be dealt with.

Indeed, even if megavitamins and orthomolecular approaches ultimately do prove to have little validity, to deprive Mrs. G of what worked for her would be tragic, unnecessary, and illogical as well. It would be to confuse overwhelming statistical predominance with absolute reality, a major category error. The importance of this issue to psychiatry can be clarified by discussing the current status of schizophrenia.

Schizophrenia, a severely disabling disorder that perverts its victims' thoughts and very sense of identity, is not yet understood, nor is there definitive treatment for more than a few isolated cases. Yet, it is a hotbed for reductionism, and provides a good example for discussing the current disarray of our professional practice. Biology is currently in the forefront, with convincing data that 50 percent of identical twins but only 15 percent of fraternal twins will share the disorder, and that the influence of those who raise the children is comparatively unimportant. May's (1968) monumental study of treatment shows that 70 percent respond to antipsychotic medication but not psychotherapy. While there are a few striking case histories of psychotherapeutic cure and an extensive family therapy literature supporting the importance of disturbed communication in the social setting, the biological evidence dominates the current thinking and is felt by many to "prove" that schizophrenia is fundamentally a biological derangement and that problems at other levels are outgrowths of this.

While these data are impressive, they do not demonstrate that the disorder is exclusively biological in nature. Fifty percent of schizophrenic identical-twin pairs are nonconcordant; thus, the biological data themselves show that other factors also must contribute. May's study shows equally convincingly that nearly 30 percent of schizophrenics respond better to psychotherapy than medication. To ignore that 30 percent is to make the error of translating statistical dominance into absolute reality — that 30 percent still amounts to many suffering patients who will be denied the help currently available if we treat them only by "majority rule." The error was not emphasizing the advances in biological understanding and treatment; rather it was the rigid linear causal thinking that led us to believe it was either-or, that if it were biological in nature, then it could not be psychological or social.

Of the 30 percent who do not respond to antipsychotic medication, some may represent a different kind of disorder altogether, like Mrs. R with her spontaneous trances (see Introduction). Others require an entirely different psychobiological formulation, like Mrs. G. In either case, the distinction between overwhelming statistical predominance and absolute reality needs to be kept in mind.

Failure to use double-blind techniques was also a major factor in the categorical rejection of orthomolecular approaches by a recent APA task force (1973), as noted by Hoffer (1974). He countered that the very nature of orthomolecular treatment was so complex and comprehensive that it could not be tested by controlling specific variables. It would require a comparison with traditional approaches *en masse*, which has yet to be carried out.

Holistic biological approaches such as comprehensive megavitamin therapy, environmental manipulation, and clinical ecology are similarly unsuited to direct experiment because of their comprehensive nature. Controlled experiment requires the teasing out of specific variables. If the comprehensiveness of the approach is what works we would expect negative results from testing isolated component variables. Similar problems plague psychotherapy research.

CASE 2. CRAZY OR CREATIVE?

Mrs. H, a 30-year-old woman in ongoing treatment for relationship problems and chronic despair, came into my office in a crisis. She fearfully revealed episodes of depersonalization, with altered body image and sensory distortions such as illusions, visual images, and altered perception of time. She added that she frequently had precognitive, telepathic, and clairvoyant experiences whose thought content frequently checked out. She was terrified that she was either crazy or might be considered so by others.

While her initial hypotheses were close to the red line, Mrs. H was still clear and coherent. She remained a bright young lady with an inquiring mind, an expansive personality competent in most aspects of everyday living. Considered by themselves, her experiences sounded more like spontaneous hypnosis similar to that of Mrs. R (see Introduction). With her having otherwise intact thought processes, I encouraged her to simply keep in mind the distinction between experiences and beliefs about them. Experiences are neither right nor wrong, true nor false, good nor bad; they simply are. By contrast, beliefs about them clearly can be true, false, or even crazy by most social and professional standards. She was advised to look at her experiences simply as interesting phenomena and to absolutely avoid facile explanations. With benevolent skepticism advised, her psychic phenomena did not interfere with social or occupational functioning nor cause her further distress; i.e., they were not unhealthy. Mrs. H has continued to progress in personal growth.

FACTUAL JUDGMENT AND THE UNTESTABLE

There are many clinical cases like Mrs. H that illustrate the importance of keeping clear where factual judgments are appropriate and where they are not. Severe cognitive psychopathology and even psychosis can result from a simple category error in factual judgment, just as so much affective distress follows from inappropriately applying moral judgments to one's basic being instead of his actions (see Table 3.2, p. 58). When beliefs about experiences are confused with the experiences themselves, they can take on that quality of subjective certitude that characterizes fixed delusions. To avoid a sense of helplessness, an important human need is to give some meaning to unusual experiences. Any biological process that subverts thought or mood is likely to create unusual experiences that will be so misinterpreted; probably an intrinsic mechanism of delusion formation in schizophrenic and affective disorders. Skilled cognitive therapy may interdict the delusional process in some cases, even while the underlying defect persists. With patients less cognitively intact than Mrs. H, it is especially important for the psychiatrist evaluating an unusual thought process to ascertain what experiences underlie the beliefs and how the patient goes from one to another.

We need to distinguish between basic existence and our beliefs about this existence. Experiences are simply internal phenomena, aspects of what is. Only beliefs are subject to factual judgment. Two errors are commonly made along this continuum of experiences and beliefs: 1) to overexplain the unexplainable, which can lead to psychosis or elaborate belief systems that few others can relate to; and 2) to confuse unexplainability with nonexistence, common in scientific practice at its highest levels.

Ken Wilber (1983) warns us against another category error that can lead to psychosis, the Pre/Trans Fallacy, or falsely equating regressive experiences with transcendent ones just because they share the common factor of being nonrational. The Pre/Trans Fallacy could lead either to discounting transcendental experiences as merely psychotic or could worsen a true psychosis by mislabeling it as transcendent.

BEYOND THE CONTROLLED EXPERIMENT

The historical fate of Anton Mesmer (Sheehan & Perry, 1976) illustrates the risk of equating "not yet explained" with "does not exist." Alarmed by the growing popularity of Mesmer's "animal magnetism" fad, the French government appointed a Commission of Inquiry to investigate his work, choosing Benjamin Franklin as its chairperson and including several noted scientific dignitaries.

The subsequent study was a paragon of the classic scientific method, a well-controlled blind experiment that conclusively proved, among other things, that a "magnetized" tree had no therapeutic effect on a patient unless the latter expected it to. The common denominator of the Commission's findings was that the theory of animal magnetism was categorically false, and that Mesmer's admittedly profound therapeutic results were simply "a matter of imagination." While a few diehards continued to practice Mesmer's approach, it faded into the background, and hypnosis did not recover any scientific stature until the Bernheim-Charcot controversy a full century later.

Two points are worth clarification: First, the classic scientific study contributed *no new information* but only tested *beliefs about* the information, which was already clear to everyone present — that Mesmer practiced certain behaviors and his patients experienced "crises" frequently followed by relief. What the experiment did was to rule out a patently absurd belief about these data that some substance or force mediated Mesmer's effects. It was the belief that was proven false, not the treatment successes, which still remain to be explained.

Second, the baby got thrown out with the bathwater, as often happens even today following scientific repudiation. Mesmer's results were a matter of "imagination"; hence, it was as if they did not exist, in violation of the positive data that actually led to the study in the first place. Had this category error not been made, the data might have been interpreted literally, anticipating the hypnosis research from the 1960s on that illustrates the pivotal role of imagination in both health and illness. To disprove a clearly untenable explanation still leaves the phenomenon unexplained.

More recently, the well-known psychic Jane Roberts (1966/1976) has described methods of systematic observation similar to those of Freud and Piaget, carefully designed to minimize the possibility of observer bias while acknowledging that it cannot be eliminated. Many of her subsequent beliefs are far-out by conventional scientific standards and far beyond scientific testing, but they dovetail with similar beliefs developed independently by other psychics with less or comparable qualifications. These include relativity of space and time, existence of "alternate realities" existing side by side along with our own, and extension of "thought" or spiritual substance beyond its usual physical bounds. While this material might ultimately prove as invalid as the animal magnetism of Mesmer, the observations themselves remain, waiting to be explained.

Physics and astronomy share these dilemmas of the untestable. Cosmology must forever remain beyond scientific testing, since there is no way we can redo the big bang in the laboratory. Such speculations are an important part of current scientific thinking, however, and they do spur on useful research by suggesting associated hypotheses. Black holes are postulated to explain otherwise anomalous data, and they suggest that the very fabric of space-time may warp and fold back on itself into "layers" of reality that could be superimposed on one another. The quantum theory, which successfully makes sense of particle physics, also implies that within any finite space is a nearly infinite amount of "zero point energy" that is not manifest (testable) but is really real (Bohm, 1971). Even classical electromagnetic theory of the vacuum yields similar results (Boyer, 1985). Bohm (1980) is reexamining the premises of modern physics to account for these and other findings. His "new order" not only allows for multiple physical dimensions, but also postulates "noncausal correlations" that bear a strong resemblance to the synchronicity of Jung, and gives a high place to consciousness in the new physics.

If much of the world of even physics and astronomy is beyond the possibility of precise measure, testing, or statistical evaluation, this is so much more the case for the human mind. A third case will illustrate a further limitation against precision in the scientific method. Even where the clinical data was accessible, it was necessary to employ two partially contradictory models in order to adequately understand and treat her presenting complaints, a paradox not uncommon in clinical practice.

CASE 3. TWO-AND-A-HALF

Ms. V was a 40-year-old woman with a long history of alcohol abuse with episodic blackouts, and chronic depression with bouts of suicidal behavior that she often did not remember. She had proven resistant to psychiatric treatment for years and stubbornly refused to address her alcohol dependency. Exploratory hypnosis subsequently confirmed a clear diagnosis of multiple personality with two well-defined part-selves entrenched in bitter internal warfare. The amnesic episodes could be understood as dissociative, with alcoholic damage putting these further and further beyond her control. The drinking could be viewed as a desperate attempt to relieve her dysphoria, as she herself maintained.

Two personalities were identified. In her "usual self" state of mind, Rita was constricted and compulsive. She slavishly sought approval while passively resisting any perceived threat to her autonomy. The secondary personality, who called herself Leslie, was energetic and outgoing, and often "came out" when intoxicated. Rita drank to quiet the conflict. Leslie drank to get free, although she preferred coming out without chemical assistance whenever possible. Leslie appeared as a classic "demon" (Beahrs, 1982b, Chapters 6 and 7): progressing from initial rage to becoming a steadfast therapeutic ally, and appearing to represent most of the patient's life energy. Through the classic approach of internal diplomacy, the two parties reached a satisfactory compromise in the definition of overall self-identity and sense of direction.

Or so it seemed. On increasing occasions the patient acted out against her new life decisions, sometimes with alcohol abuse and at other times with purposeful behavior contrary to her stated intentions. Occasionally, Rita claimed amnesia for these episodes, but at other times accepted their full responsibility without appearing to notice the contradictions involved. Her well-defined alternate, Leslie, denied any complicity and further denied that any other alter-personalities were involved. "Rita's simply a damn liar."

As the primary personality, Rita finally acknowledged "mixed feelings" about her positive decisions and that she had acted out against them on several occasions, withholding information from me to avoid disapproval. But at times she lost control over this process, especially when alcohol was involved, at which point it took on a life of its own beyond Rita's awareness and without switching to Leslie. Within this primary ego state, then, Rita alternated between fusion with willful conning and further splitting. Sometimes there were only the two personalities overall, but at other times there was another: Ms. V was a "two-and-a-half" personality.

Treatment was now at another impasse, although overall functioning was much higher than it had been at the earlier one. The alcohol abuse was now taking over the number one position in the patient's complex pathology, as it so often does whatever the origin of the disorder. Resolving conflicts between her parts was woefully inadequate for such a "whole person" issue, and she now needed to be dealt with as a hard-core alcoholic. I recommended the intensive multifaceted approach of the typical alcohol treatment unit.

We were left with the interesting situation in which two somewhat antithetical formulations and treatment approaches were required. If she was dealt with only as an alcoholic whole person, some alter-personality could sabotage treatment, as actually occurred prior to my own work with her. But if treatment was limited to working through conflicts between the parts, continued alcoholic debaucheries would preclude the integration that would appear necessary for meaningful sobriety. From the first perspective, sobriety is a precondition for all treatment, but from the second, integration is a precondition for any meaningful attempt at long-term sobriety. I recommended a well-coordinated alternation between the two.

CONSTRUCTS AND THEIR LIMITS OF RELEVANCE

Ms. V illustrates the limits of our constructs at two equally important levels, ego states and therapeutic belief systems. It was clearly not possible to specify her degree of multiplicity. She was a "two-and-a-half personality" in the sense of alternately being a dual and a triple personality with blurred boundaries, depending on her degree of awareness and control, which itself depended on her biochemical status. At the same time, two comprehensive belief systems with their associated treatment modalities were both necessary to adequately deal with her conflicting needs.

Several colleagues criticized my multiple-consciousness approach on the grounds that it required a logical fallacy, dealing with a complex set of processes as if it were an entity or thing. Similar criticism is often leveled at psychodynamic constructs like "ego," implying an organism or thing instead of a collection of active processes that serve a common function.

I have supported these constructs for two reasons (Beahrs, 1982a). First, any complex entity is simultaneously one, composed of many, and part of a greater whole. Which perspective to employ depends more on what works than actual truth. It is hard to imagine having achieved rapport with such an important part of Ms. V's personality as Leslie had we not addressed it as if an entity with its own thoughts and feelings. Second, communication requires the use of words and labels to denote whatever is to be discussed. Nominalization is thus a prerequisite for communication at all levels, from simple baby talk to the most esoteric scientific discourse.

My colleagues' criticism does not negate the concept of ego states as much as it clarifies how they are formed. If the patient treats different aspects of life as if they were truly separate, this actually creates the separation at the level of psychic reality. By acting as if he were a tennis player (Gallwey, 1976) and experiencing his "role" as congruently as possible (Sarbin & Coe, 1972), a person actually becomes a tennis player. The abstraction becomes real, and in fact, we have created our own reality through our beliefs (Roberts, 1974). Spanos (1986) presents considerable data showing that the form of hidden observers depends profoundly on the context in which they are elicited.

A similar process of concretizing the complex occurs even in the process of defining a physical entity like a chair. An entity is simply a collection of matter-energy with certain defining characteristics and boundaries that persist over a finite period of time. Living requires that we form concepts with enduring stability in the face of complexity and change, and to manipulate these with mental operations and language. From this process of compartmentalizing nature that we call language arises power for action at more than just an instinctive level. Ideally, the constructs will correspond to what they point toward in external reality, but no entity ever becomes more than a useful abstraction, an "approximation to the whole truth" (Feynman, Leighton, & Sands, 1963).

Figure 7.1 illustrates the nature of constructs and their limits. The many intersecting lines are intended to represent the complex lines

Figure 7.1. Complex causality

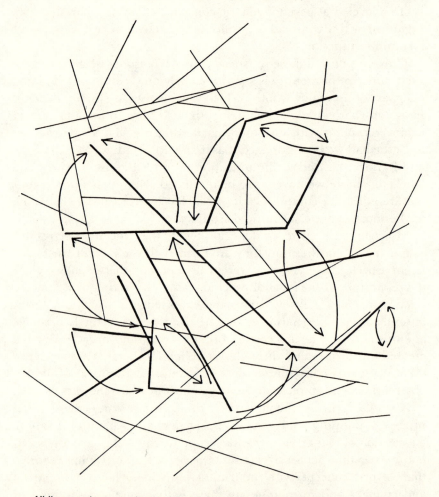

All lines and arrows denote hypothetical causal relationships
Bold lines refer only to those proposed by a specific theoretical system

of linear and circular causality in what is. The bold lines denote those causal elements specified by a particular complex construct, a therapeutic system. They illustrate where that construct is useful or relevant, its domain. The lighter lines depict causal elements not specified by the system, and lie beyond its scope. They represent elements of reality where the construct simply does not apply. "Limits of relevance" are simply those beyond which a given construct is no longer useful, where another is needed.

Figure 7.2 illustrates this in another way. The surface area depicts the collection of individuals who potentially come to psychiatric attention. Within the double lines, psychiatry's domain, are those for whom psychiatric intervention is appropriate. A person outside these limits would do better elsewhere; one in the lower left might have a physical ailment and one in the lower right some social issue, each transcending the limits of our specialty. Each subcircle defines a particular psychiatric system, like hypnosis or formal psychobiology (the outward pointing arrows indicate my belief that these two are rapidly expanding in their scope). The two smallest subcircles illustrate more specialized models within a single system, in this case, the psychodynamic (analytical) approaches.

Referring again to Figure 7.1, it is clear that the more rigidly the bold lines specify a system's proposed causal relationships, the more likely it becomes that other variables will render it invalid in a given case, thus, unreliable. Or it is adequate in only a much smaller number of cases. For this reason it is impossible to unify psychiatry under a single system that is precise, reliable, and comprehensive.

We can have the best of both worlds only by splitting up into many subsystems that each can apply only to a select subpopulation of patients. The problem becomes one of selecting the best system, and is illustrated by several specific points in the Figure 7.2.

Person A, in the center of psychiatry's domain, represents someone nearly anyone would see as in need of psychiatric help. Which modality to choose is problematic, however. He falls into the scope of such diverse approaches as hypnosis and psychobiology and might do adequately in either. He would be problematic within psychoanalysis, however, and two of its submodels would be entirely inappropriate. Person B would not do well in psychiatry at all, falling nearly at its limits. He might even do better outside of psychiatry altogether, possibly by getting involved in some social action cause that gives him a sense of purpose and direction.

Worse yet, Ms. V illustrates the fact that even a single individual may not be dealt with adequately using any one system alone, but may require two or more formulations with mutually contradictory elements. For example, she needed treatment for primary alcoholism,

Figure 7.2. Domains and limits of relevance

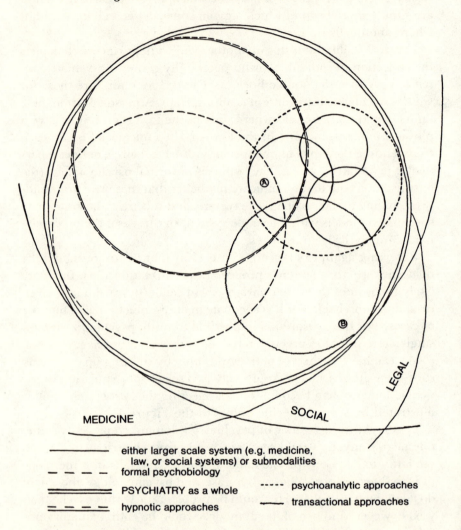

but dissociative disorder contravened. She also needed a hypnotically based neodissociative approach, but here the alcoholism was likely
to contravene. Each is a precondition for the other to be reasonably
effective.

The triage function, determining what system to refer a patient for
full evaluation and treatment, should become the task of the evaluating
psychiatrist more than it currently is in clinical practice. Since no doc-

tor can become expert at all modalities that might be used, his broad training can ideally expose him to enough of their essential features and limits so he can then refer a patient more competently to where he is most likely to benefit. This is the art of differential therapeutics, to be discussed further in Chapter 8.

THE SCIENTIFIC METHOD: COMPLEX, INTEGRATED, AND LIMITED

Kuhn (1962/1970) has presented a unified view of how science evolves from one paradigm to others. Each has a limited validity compatible with the data base of its time and becomes more inadequate as this data base grows. Acceptance of the prevailing paradigm is followed by a period of turmoil and professional self-doubt, until a new paradigm is achieved that is better able to synthesize the new data. The scientific paradigm is like a world view that *contracts* our expanding knowledge into manageable concepts, by excluding that which is irrelevant. It is an attempt to force nature into a box. We experience greater control and some relief from uncertainty with its associated sense of infantile helplessness. Ultimately, as Rothstein (1980) maintains, this adds a narcissistic investment that gives our world views so much power. In clinical practice, it allows the practitioner to "face the uncertainty" of his clinical work by mitigating it.

Rothstein warns of several disadvantages of this narcissistic investment. Overvaluing a given idea isolates its proponents from colleagues with differing ideas, and a proponent frequently presents his paradigm as "the *only* organizing framework" for clinical data. This relates to cultism and its inseparability from scientific innovation.

In summary the scientific method should be considered as encompassing three separate processes: the creative hunch, systematic observation, and the controlled experiment (see Fig. 7.3). Since the first pervades all human and probably all animal life, I will limit use of the word *scientific* to only the latter two processes, which must occur either together or one after the other, in either case with a constant give-and-take of information.

The first scientific process is systematic observation, a searchlight focused on a particular area of human endeavor whose focus is already determined by the nonrational elements described. Observation must be systematic and as unbiased as possible, its purpose being to accu-

Figure 7.3. The scientific method

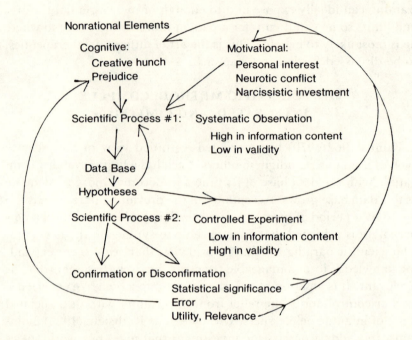

mulate, and not to evaluate, data. Only when a vast body of data is obtained do *patterns* then become evident, leading to theories such as those of Freud, Piaget, and Roberts, as well as ideas like the big bang and black holes. Giving greater scientific credibility to this process is the fact that pattern recognition is itself becoming a rigorous sub-discipline of mathematics (Tou & Gonzalez, 1974).

Only when tentative beliefs are well formed does the second scientific process, the controlled experiment, become useful. Here a hypothesis is formulated and an experimental situation constructed so that the belief can be tested, proven either true or false, relevant or irrelevant, useful or not, as the case may be. The scientific method does not end here, as the results of an experiment will shed light on our beliefs, force modifications, and raise new questions that will ultimately stimulate new emotional needs, help focus our searchlight in different directions, and possibly even suggest new areas for data collection as well as experiment. Ultimately, science is *knowing*, and includes both the rational and nonrational elements of knowledge.

8

The Differential
Therapeutic Index

OVERVIEW

Differential therapeutics is the art and science of treatment selection (Frances, Clarkin, & Perry, 1984). It should include not only the choice of specific interventions, but also the process of determining by which psychiatric system or modality a patient is best conceptualized and treated; that is, which framework provides for that particular patient the most clear understanding of his problems, and the greatest likelihood of efficient and effective treatment results. This choice of system can be called the Differential Therapeutic Index or DTI. I propose that psychiatric systems in current use be codified, and that the Differential Therapeutic Index be amended to a patient's clinical diagnosis. For DSM-III, the DTI would be an Axis VI. This chapter will review the factors leading to this recommendation and discuss the type of clinical reasoning involved in making such a treatment-oriented diagnosis.

Most therapists require a fairly well-defined theoretical structure in order to guide their work and provide protection. But it is not possible, even in principle, to unify all of mental health under a single comprehensive system that is precise enough to predicate the many refined technical interventions at our profession's disposal, and is reliable enough to ensure reasonable confidence in the outcome. A precise system can be reliable only within a small portion of our profession's domain. Hence, it is unavoidable that our profession will be fragmented into many competing systems, frameworks, or modalities that cannot be reduced to one another. To make the most of this state of affairs is the task with which differential therapeutics is charged: If multiple psychiatric systems are like orchestra members, we need to find a conductor.

Scientific parameters alone are not enough for this choice since it is often the "untestable intangibles" that prove to be the determining factor. These are a major reason that another axis needs to be amended to the clinical diagnosis. Two large-scale social trends in mental health are contributing toward this goal: 1) a move toward specifying all treatment parameters with more scientific precision; and 2) a move toward respecting the uniqueness of every individual. To a large extent these two trends work against one another.

The first trend, toward more precise scientific specification, dates back over two decades to when Watkins (1960) outlined the many psychotherapies in vogue at that time, attempting to clarify their indications and contraindications. Putting differential therapeutics on solid scientific ground has received increased attention more recently. Frances, Clarkin, and Perry (1984a) summarize the current state of the art, following on the heels of two APA-supported surveys (Karasu, 1984; Lewis & Usdin, 1982). Lazarus (1981) had earlier incorporated multiple biopsychosocial parameters into his own specific "multimodel" modality, and the prevailing paradigm in all of psychiatry is the biopsychosocial model of Engel (1980). Diagnosis-related treatment specificity is also part of this trend, with even more recent attempts having been made to systematize the psychotherapy of depression (Klerman, Weissman, Rounsaville, & Chevron, 1985) and anxiety (Beck & Emery, 1985). All of these contributions represent an increasing attempt by scientific psychiatry to systematize its domain and specify its parameters.

The second, concurrent trend is a move away from diagnosis-related specificity, toward a belief that all patients must be dealt with as unique individuals. Some Ericksonian therapists, for example, believe that *any* precisely defined therapeutic system is a Procrustean straightjacket to be avoided at all costs. If psychotherapy is truly formulated to meet the uniqueness of the individual's needs, then perhaps referral into any fixed or defined system of beliefs and techniques would be too limiting. If so, perhaps all such systems should become obsolete, in which case a differential therapeutic index would become either meaningless, or just a palliative for an unacceptable state of affairs.

My own position is in between: increasing scientific precision and respecting human uniqueness are two processes that must coexist and that cannot be fully reconciled to one another. On the one hand, each limits the other's scope, but on the other hand, ensures that it will be employed only where most appropriate.

Diagnosis-related specificity is limited in a fundamental way by the many untestable intangibles of the psychological level that determine human uniqueness and that underlie the roots of uncertainty in mental health. For example, one overly rigid compulsive patient might welcome permission for more spontaneity, but another might resist any attempts at being "loosened up" with all his might. The second might respond better to defining and adhering to his value structure even more, with the result that he feels safer from himself and is able to allow himself more flexibility and spontaneity as a by-product. This may be determined by quirks of human language outside of what can be specified. And similar value connotations can determine whether or not to use antidepressants to treat a depressed individual. If a biological formulation helps the patient save face, this will add to the medication's effect, but if it makes him feel defective the effect may be negated.

What is true at one level may be false or irrelevant at another. Similarly, a person may have chosen something at one level that "just happens" at another, rendering it impossible to precisely and reliably determine whether or not he chose and is thus responsible for his actions.

The chains of complex linear and circular causality, at multiple biological, psychological, and social levels are so intricate that, inevitably, any theory will leave out something that might be important. The task of science and scientific therapy is to draw out those key features that can be changed. But the more precisely we specify those parameters, the more likely it is that they will be inconsistent or irrelevant, thus unreliable. This is the essence of the uncertainty principle in mental health.

There is an even more obvious limit to the second trend, the one moving towards greater individualization. Few therapists are capable of unstructured flexibility without unconscionable sacrifice of protectiveness. While structure can certainly be like a straightjacket, it is also essential in avoiding chaos by providing an orderly sense of direction, methodology, and protective grounding. Even Erickson's legendary flexibility was not based on lack of a system, framework or structure; he just kept his beliefs to himself. I summarized (Beahrs, 1982a) my understanding of his system as: a basic faith in fundamental reality; an unswerving integrity based on fairly conservative values; a "commonsense psychology" and awareness that this was occurring simultaneously at multiple levels that could be communicated with even when "hidden"; a clear sense of priorities; a keen sense of the multiple polar opposites; and the ability to positively reframe most life events thereby gaining control of and a direction in life. It would be misleading to say that this is not a system; it is one, a system of beliefs that need scientific testing as much as any other.

We are now back where we started. Structure is necessary to provide direction and protection to our work, yet no structure can be precise, reliable, and comprehensive. We can have the best of both worlds, however, if we embrace more than one psychiatric system, using each only where relevant. While no precise system can embrace more than a small fraction of specific cases, it is equally true that rare is a specific case problem for which *some* precise model cannot be reliably applied. If collectively the narrow but precise models can largely encompass the human condition, then having access to each part of the whole affords us the potency of technique and the specificity of understanding that each model provides within its limited domain. Our profession can have the advantages of specialization or division of labor, that which has always favored complex organisms in the course of evolution.

The task becomes that of organization and selection. For there to be any reliable way of selecting which model to call forth for a specific case problem, there must be some overall executive belief system encompassing the multiple modalities in a less precise but more inclusive umbrella. Lack of this comprehensive umbrella underlies the occasional chaotic infighting in our profession. We are like a disturbed multiple personality; perhaps an approach similar to integrating a multiple personality into a "union of many states" will be useful to integrating the mental health profession as well. The roadblocks are similar in the two cases: There are no rules of procedure for determining whose claim to the executive role is legitimate, and there may be more than one way. The approach inevitably becomes pragmatic.

ROADBLOCKS TO
DIFFERENTIAL THERAPEUTICS

To develop a differential therapeutic index, or treatment-oriented diagnosis, we need to develop criteria for use of a particular system or modality. To do this we also need to systematically study a variety of psychiatric frameworks, continually seeking to define their domains or limits of relevance. What does each modality claim? What does each actually do, and if this is different from what is claimed, in what way? Who benefits and who is harmed by a given modality, and in what way? What can each system contribute to increased understanding of what human life is all about, as well as to more potent treatment of life's many problems? What is the role of this system in relation to that of others and to the body of human knowledge overall?

One roadblock to differential therapeutics is linguistic — we tend to use the word *modality* in different ways. Originally, it referred to a well-defined technical procedure employed to reach a clear-cut goal, as in the use of penicillin to treat streptococcal infections. Antipsychotic and antidepresant medication, ECT, and some clearly circumscribed behavioral and cognitive therapies can be understood in these terms. With words like *psychoanalysis* and *transactional analysis*, however, an additional element may supercede. These are not techniques per se, but complex theoretical and therapeutic systems based on assumptions of limited validity that include many treatment techniques within their domains. Yet we still use the term *modality*, and differential therapeutics must respect this common usage.

Hypnosis is at yet another level. It is not, like psychoanalysis or TA, a theory or even a complex set of theories. Rather, it is a set of *phenomena*, of behaviors and experiences that we do not fully understand but that are nearly universal, have profound therapeutic implications, and that any theoretical system must address and deal with if it is to be adequate. Yet the word *hypnosis* is used not only as if it were just one of many theoretical approaches, but also as if it were a technical procedure like a surgical operation or a shot of Thorazine[R]

All three senses of the word modality share what Jerome Frank (1973) considers essential to all therapy: *a setting, a trusting relationship with a competent benevolent authority, a rationale, and a treatment method thought to be based on the rationale.* He did not discount those factors unique to specific modalities, but simply asserted that we lack sufficient information to know whether modalities help people the way their proponents think they do, or to know who is best treated by whom and in which circumstances. He suggested that these questions be heavily researched. Whatever the sense in which we are using *modality*, this is the task posed for the Differential Therapeutic Index.

Another trouble spot will be what the place is for the unusual or unorthodox, such as the orthomolecular modalities, which some see as a new paradigm but others write off as a fad or cult with no objective validity. A similar dilemma is unorthodox uses of accepted modalities, such as lithium for personality disorders or hypnotic imagery for cancer victims. To be truly workable, differential therapeutic criteria must fulfull simultaneously two sometimes-opposing tasks: 1) to protect patients against the ravages of outright quackery or of undisciplined faddism, which is so often a defensive fit focusing on a part at the expense of the whole, facilitating avoidance; and 2) to allow and even encourage the use of innovative treatment modalities both to increase our fund of knowledge and to offer difficult patients the maximum benefits that our profession — even at its very fringes — can offer.

My preference was stated in Chapter 6: to use a "therapeutic presumption" similar to criminal law's innocent until proven guilty. Here, the presumption would be in favor of the standard of the accepted practice in the community. The burden of proof is on the one who favors an unusual approach, to show that what orthodox treatment offers is unacceptable, that his alternative holds at least the possibility of a more desirable outcome, and that the hazards would be low enough to retain a positive benefit/detriment analysis. Creativity would be preserved, but in a more protective manner.

Such benefit/detriment analyses will ultimately come down to value judgments that cannot be resolved by scientific criteria. In addition, intertherapist variability even within the same modality is so great that, in principle, therapists as well as modalities would need to be classified. For these and similar reasons, there is little to either hope or fear that differential therapeutics could become so refined as to be "cookbook," and hamper the creative flexibility that should remain a hallmark of the effective psychiatrist and psychotherapist.

The more precisely we define our criteria, the more they become subject to violation and absurdity. Yet if the proposed guidelines can help us head our patients in the right direction in even a general sense, that will free the choice of modality from the near-random guesswork or dependence on the evaluating psychiatrist's prejudices on which it has been all too often dependent in the past — no mean feat. Then, when it is up to the treating professional's creativity, it will at least be a professional whose specialized training is in the area most likely to be of special benefit to that particular patient.

THE PROCESS OF DIFFERENTIAL THERAPEUTICS

An appropriate differential therapeutic index is the modality by which a clinical situation is best conceptualized and treated. It must satisfy five basic criteria (see Table 8.1):

1) It provides a clear, accurate, and parsimonious explanation of the patient's difficulties, helping these to fall into place for patient and doctor alike, and provides a clear data base from which to derive treatment strategies;
2) the formulation not only makes sense to the patient, but also supports his pride and self-esteem, enhancing motivation. Creative face-saving is an aspect of this not to be minimized;
3) it provides a clear rationale for treatment interventions that can be directed at (a) *primary causality*, when such is demonstrable and accessible to treatment, (b) *focal points*, whose effects will then extend to other levels as well, (c) a multimodel *"working through,"* or when none of these options are available, (d) *palliatives*, whose benefit/detriment ratios are acceptable;
4) the ideal of mental health, as conceptualized by the modality, provides an appropriate corrective for the patient's particular pathology, as opposed to supporting a defensive avoidance, or simply being irrelevant; and
5) no contraindications are present, such as unacceptable biological, psychological, or social side effects.

TABLE 8.1
Criteria for Differential Therapeutic Index

A. *Inclusion Criteria: Appropriate Treatment Modality*
1. Accurate, parsimonious explanatory value is provided by the modality's basic assumptions.
    a) makes sense to patient and therapist alike
2. Supports patient's pride, self-esteem, sense of OKness
3. Provides rationale for intervention strategies, directed in decreasing priority toward
    a) primary causality
    b) focal points
    c) working through
    d) palliative relief:
        i. — normalization (e.g. antidepressant medication, felt to correct underlying abnormal condition).
        ii. — compensation (e.g. sedatives, which only counteract a target symptom).
4. Ideal of mental health is appropriate corrective
    a) no defensive fits
    b) no irrelevant fits
5. Absence of contraindications

B. *Exclusion Criteria: Inappropriate Treatment Modality*
1. Inordinate complexity
    a) Explanatory formulations become cumbersome, unwieldy and self-contradictory, violating the A/Not-A absurdity.
    b) speculative "fine adjustments" need to be employed to deal with anomalies.
2. Threatens patient's self-esteem
    a) patient feels misunderstood
    b) exaggerates shame and guilt
    c) leads to demoralization, with impaired motivation
3. Problematic effects
    a) increased resistance
    b) no response
    c) problematic side effects, beyond the expected
4. Ideal of mental health is antithetical to patient's needs (e.g. the self responsibility of Gestalt, for a narcissistic personality with already too little appreciation of his impact on others)
5. Clear contraindication present
    a) unacceptable side effects
       negative benefit/detriment analysis
    b) another modality more effective and/or efficient for same function

---

There should not be another modality that will serve the same functions more expeditiously than the one at hand. When two or more appropriate modalities are not redundant, however, they can and often should be employed. There will then be two or more DTIs, listed in order of decreasing priority.

The process of differential therapeutics is simply competent orthodox psychiatric practice with special attention given to the intangibles that influence a patient's attitudes and that are not addressed by scientific theory, in order to best serve the patient's needs. It requires a nearly continual assessment of data flowing in from many sources, what I refer to as the "multifactorial reevaluation," a cornerstone of the Differential Therapeutic Index and illustrated in Figure 8.1.

Figure 8.1. Matrix for differential therapeutics

	Causality, Points of Intervention			
Psychiatric Diagnosis	Primary Causality	Vicious Circles Focal Points	Palliatives	Multifactorial Re-evaluation
Psychological: identity direction conflicts values history		DIFFERENTIAL		Response to initial interventions
Biological: medical & family history response to treatments		THERAPEUTIC		New Data biological psychological social
Social: cultural & spiritual identity family control		INDEX		Consider unusual modalities
	Frame of Reference	Logical Categories	Negative Fits	
		Patient as a Person		

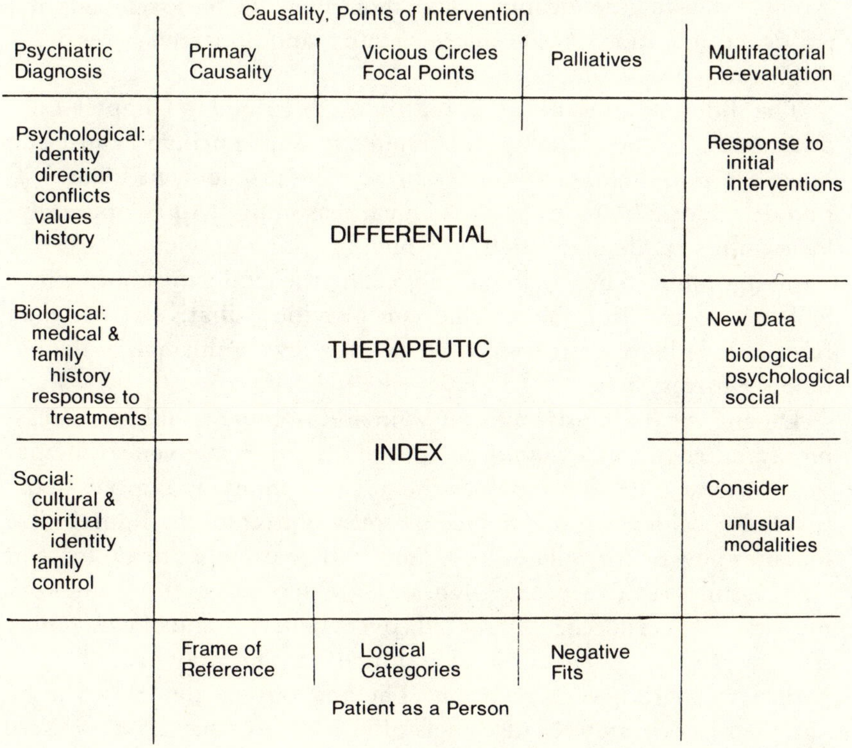

The first step is a full psychiatric diagnosis, including the psychological, biological, and social aspects of the evaluation as outlined on the left side of the figure. Within the traditional format, the psychiatrist pays the utmost attention to the patient's sense of personal *identity*: who he is, what he stands for, his wish and value priorities and any conflicts surrounding these. An important aspect of identity is *sense of direction*, not only flowing from the past into the present, but also toward a *future* that we hope to impact. The contrast between what a patient *wants* and *expects* for his future may give us information most critical for modality choice, not available from present status and past history alone. Biological identity is equally important; medical status, body style and physical habits, and response to prior interventions. Family history is essential to clarify constitutional factors that can determine such psychological basics as temperament and character style. Social identity, which includes how a patient's symptoms affect his family and associates, may clarify power dynamics without which his symptoms have little meaning. This should include basic religious and political orientation, socioeconomic status, and preferred styles of social intercourse.

The different types of causal reasoning described in Chapter 1 are outlined at the top of the figure. When a treatable primary cause can make sense of the patient's entire presenting problem, its identification demands a high priority in clinical reasoning. More commonly, focal points can be identified, of which breaking up vicious circles is most common. When these are not clear, the clinician should either look for aggravating factors that can provide palliative relief when removed, or be prepared for an in-depth working through of the patient's entire system.

During the diagnostic interview, in addition to careful risk assessment and cognitive evaluation, special attention is given to the patient's frame of reference, which includes the many intangibles of the psychological level and is depicted on the bottom of the figure. This includes how he formulates his beliefs and goals, what he omits, and how he supports his sense of OKness. Close scrutiny of this framework may identify certain deeply rooted covert beliefs, some of which may play key roles in perpetuating his difficulties and may provide focal points for cognitive intervention. The appropriate modality will be one whose own underlying beliefs offer a potent corrective to those of the patient.

In contrast to the appropriate corrective are two types of "negative fits," in which the modality's framework is compatible with the patient's, but in a counterproductive manner — a relative contraindication to the modality. The first is a "defensive fit," which supports a patient's avoidance and may perpetuate or even worsen his pathology. A clear example is the appeal of cultlike therapies to borderline personalities, in providing quick relief from their dysphoria and an easy answer. Everything seems to fall into place, but the relief is only illusory, and works against the patient truly facing the extent of his primitive despair, without which true maturation and growth are impossible. The logic of the defensive fit is that of the half-truth; it is true as far as it goes, but it is only part of the story. More often than not, it is what is omitted that does the damage. The corrective may be to abandon the modality or to add an appropriate balancing factor to reverse the defensive avoidance.

The second type is the "irrelevant fit," in which the essential cause or focal point is simply ignored. A patient may present with classic anxiety disorder, for example, with dynamics so clear and obvious that the future course of long-term psychotherapy seems entirely predictable (cf. Coffee Addict, Chapter 2). However, the patient returns a week later, having followed his physician's advice to discontinue his three pots of coffee per day, and the "obvious" dynamics are no longer present — he is cured. Had the caffeine abuse not been identified and corrected, the best of psychotherapy would have been irrelevant. Similar is the chronic psychotic whose "schizophrenia" disappears when a long-standing myxedema is reversed by thyroid replacement. Similar contrasts occur between psychological levels alone. Our main protection against this all-too-frequent type of error is to keep our minds open to as many levels as possible, to be aware of our own personal biases, and to keep open to alternative explanations.

With all of these data now at hand, the psychiatrist makes a clinical diagnosis using standard nomenclature, and formulates his initial treatment plan using the accepted method that he believes will best relieve the patient's presenting problem with the fewest side effects. At this point he should be able to specify all five axes of DSM-III, thus satisfying the current demands of clinical diagnosis. But the patient may not respond to treatment or the treatment may be accompanied by side effects nearly as severe as the presenting problem itself. In clinical practice, this is the psychiatric equivalent to a fully controlled experiment: Original hypotheses are tested, and when they prove to be problematic, new ones are needed. In addition to no response and problematic side effects, further criteria for an inappropriate modality follow from not adequately respecting the patient's own frame of reference. The inappropriate frame of reference often makes little sense to the patient, who then feels misunderstood or "put down." If he associates the modality's explanations with negative value judgments of "defective," "not-OK," etc., resistance is apt to be intense and stubborn, and in this light may seem more like an appropriate assertion of autonomy. The more that resistance is based on transference and communication factors as opposed to realistic life dilemmas, the more one should consider an alternative modality. What feels supportive to one patient feels derogatory to another. One patient is relieved by a biological explanation while another feels discounted; one feels more "understood" by an analytic formulation while another feels like he is being dissected. This can be true for patients who differ only in their frame of reference, which cannot be predicted by the usual hard medical-psychiatric data.

Making the clinical diagnosis and employing the accepted treatment methods is not sufficient for the formal DTI, the sixth axis I am proposing, since so many patients with identical descriptive diagnoses will differ dramatically in the choice of psychiatric modality most useful to understand and treat their problems. This is the main point of this entire volume. This additional axis must await the response to the initial treatment interventions, and if there is none, or if the response is problematic or the treatment inappropriate, then the continuing process of multifactorial reevaluation must be used.

When theoretical explanations become more and more cumbersome and unwieldy, and more fine adjustments need to be made, it is also time to consider an alternative system to bring to bear on the situation. An example is one in which psychoanalytic descriptions seem vague, diffuse, and circular, but the simple P-A-C of transactional analysis scores a bulls-eye in helping everything seem simple. But for a comparable patient, TA might lead to a complicated second-order "Child in the Parent of the Child" formulation, more simply understood as an Oedipal conflict. No system can cover all the bases. Most important, the clinician should cycle again and again through the type of reasoning described in this section. Diagnosis and treatment are always an ongoing process.

CASE ILLUSTRATION AND FLOW SHEET

Figure 8.2 presents a flow sheet to further guide the clinician in the process of treatment-oriented diagnosis that I am recommending. It is modeled closely after the decision trees in DSM-III (American Psychiatric Association, 1980), especially the one for psychotic disorders. I must emphasize that the flow sheet depicts only one small aspect of the complex type of multilevel clinical reasoning that is going on continually, and requires many years of professional training for its development. Most important is the history and physical examination format. At the same time the clinician will have already

Figure 8.2. Differential therapeutics flow sheet

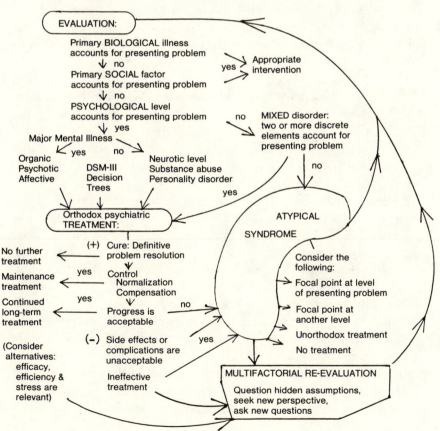

formed initial hypotheses such as "this patient is bipolar manic unless proven otherwise," which will guide and direct further inquiry. Flow sheets like Figure 8.2 and the ones in DSM-III are more like checklists, to help us think in a more organized manner, and make sure we have not overlooked something else that we should deal with. They provide protection against the self-perpetuating bias that our initial hypotheses could otherwise lead us into. This is clarified by further information gathering and validation, leading to a complex integrated type of thinking essentially the same as the scientific method, described in the last chapter. Nardone (1986) describes a similar process of clinical reasoning in general medicine.

Unlike DSM-III, the flow sheet for differential therapeutics is unitary, representing a type of process that can be applied to any clinical problem. It also differs in being circular instead of linear. Figure 8.2 keeps cycling back on itself, repeating the same steps over and over again until a satisfactory treatment modality is found. Only at this point does the clinician exit from the process, and even this is illusory since at any sign of trouble, he will reenter the flow.

Mrs. R, the complex case presented in the Introduction (p. xxviii), will be used to illustrate this type of reasoning. As we remember, Mrs. R had presented herself with a history of episodic psychosis, erratic unstable behavior, and vague physical symptoms that had eluded diagnosis. A thorough history and physical examination was done, and the immediate hypothesis was that her psychosis was most atypical and required a closer look.

Entering the flow sheet, the first requisite hypothesis was whether some illness at the biological level could account for her symptoms as a primary cause. With many prior medical workups having been negative, it was reasonable to conclude that this was not the case. Then came the social axis. Was she malingering for clear secondary gain, like legal compensation? Close scrutiny again ruled this out, but elements of passive control in her family were present and the possibility of a social intervention like family therapy was considered. But passive control did not adequately account for all her difficulties, since this can be an expression of many other primary problems, including medical. It was necessary to continue down the decision tree.

The third stop in the diagram, the possibility of a primary cause at the psychological level, proved to be more fruitful. To make this determination required our continuing on to several subsidiary questions shown on the left side of the diagram. The first is about major mental illness, by which I mean those psychiatric disorders that are defined in primarily psychological terms, but for which data point toward causal features and points of intervention at the biological level. Psychosis was definitely present, so it was necessary to cycle through the DSM-III decision tree for psychotic manifestations. This again required our asking the medical and social questions, and again answering in the negative.

Schizophrenia required closer scrutiny. Taking DSM-III criteria literally, Mrs. R would have met all criteria for this disorder except for the lack of *continuous* illness over any six-month period, and lack of deterioration in personality. The episodic course suggested bipolar disorder, but her psychotic thinking was not congruent with her mood. And at the next point on the decision tree, no clear paranoid delusions were present. In other words, with current psychiatric knowledge, this patient was atypical. No single syndrome accounted for her difficulties, even at the psychological level. The next step in the schema outlined on Figure 8.2 would have been to determine if two or more discrete formulations could together account for Mrs. R's symptoms, where one alone had failed. At first it seemed not, so it was necessary to cycle back to "atypical."

Only when asking myself if a suitable focal point could be found, irrespective of specific diagnosis, did I find the answer. The patient was acting as though she were hypnotized, and by taking charge of her spontaneous hypnotic behavior I was able to help her terminate her psychotic episode within twenty minutes. With the most urgent priority now under control — the psychotic behavior — Mrs. R now showed clear evidence of a personality disorder, a pattern of maladaptive behavior extending from before adulthood, which was interfering with social and occupational functioning. Her particular type was called *histrionic*. Two disorders together — histrionic personality and superimposed psychotic episodes best viewed as spontaneous hypnosis — now appeared to account for her disorder, which was dealt with appropriately.

The Differential Therapeutic Index for Mrs. R's personality disorder was classic orthodox treatment — exploratory psychodynamic relationship therapy. Her response to three years of this treatment was gratifying, and confirmed that this choice of modality had been appropriate. For the psychotic episodes only an unorthodox formulation adequately fit the clinical picture; that is, viewing her behavior as a disorder of hypnosis. The DTI here was simply therapeutic hypnosis, an accepted modality in itself but most unusual when employed as definitive treatment of a psychosis. Mrs. R clearly met the criteria for use of an unorthodox modality: the orthodoxy had nothing to offer her, an alternative formulation did prove viable, and there were no problematic side effects associated with its use.

It is important to realize that the process described above did not take any extra time, nor did it require any extra type of procedure per se. Many factors had already confirmed her atypical status: neither her symptoms nor her clinical course fit known syndromes, and her response to orthodox treatment of psychosis had been most problematic. I was able to hit the appropriate focal point easily, having had extensive prior experience with both clinical and research hypnosis. I knew the phenomena well and recognized them when I saw them, even though they were far from the context in which they are usually seen.

The initial bipartite DTI proved appropriate but insufficient. The persisting physical symptoms continued to evade diagnostic scrutiny, but remained sufficiently troublesome to demand continued attention. Only after the questions of an unusual formulation and unorthodox modality were asked again and again, did an additional DTI emerge at the biological level. This was clinical ecology, a complex medical discipline with only fringe status at the time, but that was able to provide an adequate working rationale and appropriate intervention. And Mrs. R also had a positive response to exogenous thyroid administration for reasons we can only speculate about; this was a fourth and final DTI.

Mrs. R's complete multiaxial diagnosis, using the Differential Therapeutic Index, is then as follows:

    Axis I: 1) Atypical Psychosis
            2) Psychological Factors Affecting Physical Condition
    Axis II: Histrionic Personality Disorder
    Axis III: 1) Status Post Cholecystectomy
              2) Atypical Allergy

     3) Atypical Thyroid Disorder

Axis IV: Psychosocial Stressors, Code 3, Mild (Family Stress)

 Axis V: Highest Level of Function in Prior Year, Level 1, Superior.

Axis VI: Differential Therapeutic Index:

     1) Therapeutic Hypnosis

     2) Exploratory Psychodynamic Relationship Psychotherapy

     3) Clinical Ecology

     4) Thyroid Administration

This entire volume has presented the multiple roots of uncertainty that render precise clinical diagnosis inadequate for many patients, to either fully understand them or to treat them with our current armamentarium. The Differential Therapeutic Index is simply a formal way to add the pragmatic treatment-oriented data that we need in order to treat our patients as well as we are capable of, in a manner consistent with current diagnostic tradition. Like any precise specification, the DTI will be limited. Disagreement about how different modalities are defined, partial integration of some modalities into others, and intertherapist differences all make the DTI most limited in its reliability. And continuing growth of our scientific data base will render many current models obsolete and provide new perspectives hardly imagined at the present time. But the Differential Therapeutic Index at least represents the best effort to improve the usefulness of current diagnosis and treatment by including the many roots of uncertainty into our broad biopsychosocial paradigm, utilizing these many factors even before we fully understand them.

The Epilogue, which follows, points beyond the scientific dimension of mental health to an even more fundamental personal level that science can never take away from us. This is the need to define our self-identity, sense of direction, and value priorities in the face of this uncertainty. A fundamental tension between the need for faith, force, and forgiveness puts this task forever beyond the limit of any scientific discipline.

Epilogue:

Faith, Force,

and Forgiveness

This work will close with material that clarifies the type of dilemmas with which it has dealt and points beyond our professional boundaries toward the broader domain of human living. The substrate of this discussion is the need for the three F's: *faithful* acceptance of all that is as a precondition for basic self-esteem; *forceful* effort to shape reality according to our will, equally essential for a meaningful sense of personal potency, meaning, and direction; and *forgiveness*, which points so far beyond the purely psychiatric dimension to the moral and spiritual side of human living from which we cannot extricate ourselves and should not try.

One of my favorite sayings throughout the years, a modified version of the Serenity Prayer, parallels this fundamental perspective for healthy living: God, give me the courage to accept what cannot and should not be changed, the strength to change what can and should be changed, and the wisdom to know one from the other. This plea comes as close as possible to summarizing my entire position.

Healthy living requires two antithetical principles, acceptance and nonacceptance, coexisting in tension with one another that can admit to no scientific resolution. Without faith or acceptance, the unfortunate individual or society is left with chronic depression (Beahrs, 1977a; Lowen, 1972) and abdication of power for constructive action (Roberts, 1974), which increases the risk of violence at the core of most human evil (Fromm, 1973; Tillich, 1951). But to exist in the sense meaningful for human identity is to impact the environment (Watkins, 1978). Without the power to do this, a person lacks the most vital aspect of living organisms and for all practical purposes does not even exist. An optimal forceful nonacceptance is thus as important as faith to give life meaning. Resolution of this dilemma must be determined by each individual and social group, based on priorities that only that entity can determine for itself.

Forgiveness, the third dimension of human living, well known since the time of Christ, generally has been ignored by scientific psychology. The principle of forgiveness in some sense transcends acceptance and nonacceptance while coexisting in tension with them. It transcends faith as well as logic and fairness, and in a strange way permits us to integrate all of these tensions in our own unique way.

To forgive means simply to grant pardon without harboring resentment (James, 1979). Literally, that means first giving up the right or the need to punish someone else, instead giving that person a clean slate. Second, it means giving up even the hard feelings that usually follow our having been wronged. This twofold giving up often feels like an insurmountable task, like it is simply too much to ask.

In traditional Christianity, forgiveness of His persecutors was a fundamental component of Christ's redemption of mankind through His willful sacrifice. Thinking in terms of the symbolic language of mythology and the unconscious (Donington, 1963), death means the giving up of old struggles, leading to renewed life and direction, or rebirth.

What is given up in the symbolic death that forgiveness represents is the need for vengeance; for righting old wrongs, for evening the score for painful hurts inflicted upon one's self when vulnerable and helpless. The wrongs that bind us to a wish for vengeance are generally threefold: 1) brutality, violence inflicted by others on an innocent and helpless self; 2) shaming, humiliation, or slight, where retribution becomes a matter of "honor"; and 3) taking away of something precious, indelibly associated with the integrity of selfhood, such as a love object.

Masterson (1981) is correct in believing that roots of vengeance go back to infantile helplessness. The traumatized child vows to never feel helpless again, and that he will pay back the real or imagined perpetrators of his pain when he "gets big enough." The early self develops to protect a person from infantile helplessness. Shaming or taking away from are equivalent to ripping off this armor, leaving us vulnerable; these are, therefore, the psychological equivalents of gross abuse.

The most intolerable aspect of traumatic affect is the associated *helplessness/powerlessness*, as clearly demonstrated by Terr's (1983) studies of traumatized children and the testimony of many war veterans. In the face of this trauma, the idea of routing a persecutor is sufficient antithesis to permit life to go on. And this sense of power may be lifesaving in certain desperate situations, as illustrated by a tragic poem (WTBS, 1985) that helped the besieged Russians to survive during their hour of doom during the Second World War.

> A great force has kept us alive
> For what they say is true
> They cry no longer
> For no tears could quench our burning hate
> And hate is our only cause,
> the guarantee of life,
> the cure for grief,
> the one uniting, warming and guiding cause

This bone-chilling manifesto says it all. Without the hate there is grief, and it often feels like the tears will never stop. And without the hate there is helpless vulnerability; it feels like survival is being put on the line. Literally true for the Russians under siege, it may feel equally desperate to the traumatized child within many a disturbed neurotic patient. Once betrayed, he will not take that risk again. This is the early decision, made for the sake of self-protection.

For the child, this illusory *sense* of power in the face of actual helplessness means he will redress his grievances when he "grows up." To forgive means to give up this sense of power, which feels like once again being at the mercy of overwhelming malevolent forces.

To seek vengeance is the traditional way to "right wrongs," and the very ethic of *fairness* requires it. This ethic maintains that the one who has done others wrong should be the one to do the suffering, not his innocent victims. This is simple commonsense decency based on a principle of equal rights. It is the traditional foundation of the criminal justice system. Through its institutionalization the ethic of fairness is society's policeman for morality as well as a deterrence to potential criminals and aggressors. To forgive requires giving up the need for fairness, often apparently at our own expense.

Even more basic, the quest for vengeance may become so indelibly associated with a person's sense of selfhood that it feels like a vital aspect of his basic being. As Smedes (1984) described for an individual who would not forgive, it was that he "could not live, could no longer be the person he was without his hatred; he had *become* his hatred" (p. 25). The tragedy was that "only forgiveness, the one thing he could not give . . . could have set [him] free" (p. 25). But his sense of selfhood originally arose during childhood to protect him from infantile vulnerability. To give it up would have been to sacrifice himself on the cross. That only Christ could do.

But the ethic of fairness is a mixed blessing. Tragic literature and opera dovetail in showing the paradox of vengeance; how it generally turns against the self and destroys it, often by what appear to be subtle twists of irony. Theologians, psychoanalysts, and psychics all have cited destructiveness stemming from powerlessness as a root of the worst human evil (Fromm, 1973; Roberts, 1974; Tillich, 1951). Hate binds a person to the hated object both logically and emotionally. Without it, the object is often not even relevant. What gives us an illusory sense of power also enslaves us, giving the hated object power and stature in our lives that it does not deserve. As Smedes (1984) puts it, "our hatred is a compliment, in a strange sort of way. The hated person is set apart from other creatures and honored as a free person" (p. 24).

Vengeance also perpetuates the original helplessness by denying it. Traumatic affect is split off or pushed aside, often with the aid of the false power of righteous vengeance-seeking. This temporarily preserves healthy function in conflict-free areas, but only at the cost of the problem never being resolved. Worse, the tyranny does not stop there. The walled-off affect is so intense and global that large sectors of one's basic being need to be denied as well. These turn back upon the self, demanding recognition and perhaps exacting their own pound of flesh from the tyrant who disowned them (Beahrs, 1982b, Chapter 7, Case 2). Where sense of selfhood is based on this process, the real self is denied. This is probably the best way to understand the concept of "false" self, discussed earlier.

Fighting for fairness may be equally destructive. Citing the increased inhumanity and destructiveness of our modern idealistic wars, Reinhold Niebuhr (1935/1956) laments that "there is no deeper pathos in the spiritual life of man than the cruelty of righteous people" (p. 203).

Vengeance is a bad bargain at all these levels. The power perpetuates the powerlessness; the righteousness perpetuates the evil; and denial of the basic realities of one's self condemns the person to the continuing hell of these realities. This parallels Faust's classic bargain with the devil.

To achieve health requires that these Faustian needs be given up. "This dynamic has lain at the core of the symptomatology of every borderline patient I have treated. He wants primarily revenge, to get back — not to get better. . . . the patient must make a choice between getting back or getting better. He cannot have both. As long as his aggression is channeled into revenge, it is not available to build psychic structure" (grow up) (Masterson, 1981, p. 188).

Forgiveness is also good reality testing. The reality is that we *are* helpless and vulnerable no matter how much we armor and protect ourselves. The economy could collapse, the sun might explode, crime is everywhere. To not take risks is to not live. More important yet, life *is* unfair whether we like it or not. Bad things happen to good people and evildoers alike, and people are born with assets and liabilities that they did nothing to deserve. Worse yet, what has happened happened, and cannot be undone. To seek vengeance upon God Himself is the ultimate in futility, and to attempt to remold reality according to our ideals is to deny what is.

To forgive is to heal this futile struggle. Smedes (1984) makes his most eloquent statement in this regard: "Forgiving is love's revolution against life's unfairness. When we forgive, we ignore the normal laws that strap us to the natural law of getting even and, by the alchemy of love, we release ourselves from our own painful pasts" (p. 94). Spinoza (1677/1951) was well aware of these issues, arguing: "He who lives under the guidance of reason, endeavors as far as possible, to render back love or kindness, for other men's hatred, anger, contempt, etc., toward him" (p. 220).

What is logical in concept is still not easy in practice. Many a patient will be stuck at this point: He may fully realize the perversity of his need to right the wrongs of the world and rebuild it in his image. He may crave in the depth of his soul the ability to forgive, if not forget, but no matter how hard he tries he is unable to let go, and keeps returning into the abyss. Two additional ironies may be conspiring against him: awareness of his own real/imagined guilt and certain practicalities of social ethics.

Guilt rarely fails to accompany righteous vindictiveness, especially in the small child whose trauma is complicated by the belief that he himself may have committed grievous wrongs and deserves punishment. Along with this is the even more devastating emotion of shame regarding the sense that he is somehow defective and inadequate. As we have seen, a destructive side effect of the "illness" model in psychiatry may be to relieve guilt only by perpetuating shame.

Four factors feed into dysfunctional guilt:

1) To avoid feeling helpless, a child may falsely "remember" events subsequent to a trauma as if they actually had happened before it (involuntary time-skewing), leading him to believe that he was responsible since he failed to prevent something of which he had foreknowledge (Terr, 1983). Anything but feeling helpless! Smith (1982) reports that "assertion of personal responsibility [where lacking in reality] is an attempt to overcome overwhelming feelings of powerlessness and helplessness in the face of the disaster" (p. 1029), even though this can "contain seeds of future turmoil" (p. 1029).
2) Where seduction was involved, the siren of old pleasures and regressive fantasies continually beckons one to return to the scene. The child usually senses at a deep level that this is perverse.
3) Disowning important aspects of one's self in itself is an act of violence, also sensed at important levels.
4) Being human, he most likely has done some things deserving of realistic guilt. These are complicated by the magical thinking that often links murderous fantasies to actual deaths in an inappropriate but nonetheless vivid manner.

For these reasons, forgiving is rarely possible without accepting forgiveness. With the controversial ethics of the Vietnam war still in our memories, expiation of guilt has an immediacy for its veterans not so prominent in the emotional causalities of prior "good" wars. And the "extent of personal blame victims accord themselves and the quality of the moral judgments they pass on their actions influence the course of the recovery process (negatively) they will follow far more than the objective severity of the stress which individuals undergo" (Smith, 1982, p. 1030).

If to accept forgiveness is often a necessary part of being able to forgive, it is opposed by equally formidable forces. These fall under the category of false pride, or narcissism. Pride and vengeance go hand in hand, as in so much tragic drama where vengeance is sought for the sake of honor. Pride and vengeance are nearly one and the same. As with vengeance, pride means never being vulnerable or ashamed again. Under the seductive guise of ethics, it perpetuates the pathogenic split within us by denying both our weak and our shady sides. As Miller (1979/1981) said, depression and grandiosity have much in common. Like the need to get back, the need to support a prideful self-image is often too much to give up.

The traditional path to forgiveness is confession, repentance, and atonement — the opposite of pride and fairness. "Repentance is the only honest entree to forgiveness" (Smedes, 1984, p. 89). We realize that "we are not really as innocent as we felt when we were first hurt. And we do not usually have a gigantic monster to forgive; we have a weak, needy, and somewhat stupid human being" (Smedes, 1984, p. 104).

Atkinson and Swizegood (personal communication, 1983) call our attention to a third component, a need to make *restitution*: doing for others to make up for a wrong that cannot be undone, unselfishly giving to others while expecting nothing back. The last part is the hitch and it requires the same "benevolent hypocrisy" necessary for creative face-saving: we are charged to give up our own pride, while respecting that of others as inviolable. The basic reason is the same: Not only is it decency, but it puts the power where it actually is, in the person who can move his own body but not that of others. Making restitution is often an important step in psychotherapy — many Vietnam veterans progress through the ranks from patient to leader of Vet Center groups and many former alcoholics similarly become alcohol counselors.

Forgiveness requires a colossal act of faith, and is an act of courage beyond comparison. It requires a selfless giving up of old protectors, a willingness to take risks, and to feel, and in many ways totally be at the mercy of, the powers that be. Ideally, one willingly allows himself to be vulnerable again, only paradoxically to feel stronger than ever. One sacrifices his need for fairness, but finds that the world seems as if by magic to be a better place — even more fair. He gives up his sense of self only to find it stronger than ever at a new level. But these results are not guaranteed and are not entirely in the person's own hands. The risk is most real.

This gets back to the idea of *love*, which Freud (1921/1979) likened to hypnosis. Both involve a loss of boundaries, extending one's own psychological selfhood to include a love object, but with the result that the self may become stronger than ever. Love and vulnerability certainly go hand in hand, and only love can conquer hate, a concept well known to the ancients. Niebuhr (1935/1956) is certainly right in his statement of "love as forgiveness" (p. 201).

But the complications do not end here. Several societal ramifications muddy the waters. First, LaHaye and Phillips (1982) point out the truism that to forgive in the face of continuing evil actions by others is simply to be a patsy. Second, to forgo appropriate anger as the "executive power of human decency" (Smedes, 1984, p. 108) or the "policeman" of human relationships (Tavris, 1982) is to invite chaos. There is simply too much real evil in the world. It is not in human nature to knuckle under without a fight, even if the fight so often worsens it and creates new evil. Even the theologian Niebuhr (1935/1956) acknowledges that "forgiveness in an absolute sense is . . . an impossibility" (p. 206). Pretensions otherwise would simply be the false pride that fosters the "tendency towards the demonic which imparts such pathos to all human history" (p. 206).

Optimal *non*acceptance, a forceful attempt to confront what we perceive as evil and change "what can and should be changed" is essential. Forgiveness as the "wisdom" of the Serenity Prayer is as limited as the first two principles even while to a degree it integrates and transcends them. But at least the "spirit of forgiveness" (Niebuhr, 1935/1956, p. 206) is possible. "The ultimate paradox of a genuine theism is that only its supramoral pinnacle is able to save its moral values from degeneration" (p. 207).

While this transcendent loss of face, or commitment to live and love fully, may be the most essential thing a patient needs to do to get better, this is more clearly than anything else something that no psychiatrist can do for him. And I believe that it is inappropriate for a psychiatrist to even try. This would be the ultimate violation of the patient's own boundaries, depriving him of that most fundamental of all human needs: to be a responsible free agent, accountable for his own choices. Love cannot be coached, and to tell another individual to give up his protectors is likely to backfire. Only the patient can know his inner needs sufficiently to know when and how to protect, and when and how much to trust.

We do much better to stay within the boundary of benevolent hypocrisy that is just decent living. We know that a patient needs to give up his pride, but instead permit him to save face, paradoxically making his task easier. We know that a patient needs to let go of pathological protectors, but we steadfastly maintain our assurance that protection is and must remain the number one priority when levels conflict. Paradoxically, the patient now feels safer to take risks on his own.

We have reached the limits of scientific psychiatry. By respecting this and the many other fundamental limits, we have actually become a stronger profession, better able to positively impact the course of human history.

Appendix:

The Uncertainty Principle

in Mental Health

OVERVIEW

The theme of this entire book has been the roots and implications of uncertainty in mental health. This appendix presents a concise formal argument for an uncertainty principle in mental health, summarizing its logical form and its essential roots and implications, for the reader who is interested in the underlying logic and in subjecting the associated hypotheses to the test of empirical research. I earlier termed this the "psychic uncertainty principle," drawing an analogy to Heisenberg's uncertainty principle in quantum physics (Beahrs, 1982b, Appendix I). To further illustrate the role of uncertainty in the specific domain of mental health as opposed to the physical sciences, I will clarify more fully how this principle differs from uncertainty in the domain of quantum physics, as well as being similar to it.

As originally presented, psychic uncertainty refers to a fundamental limitation within the domain of mental health against even the possibility that we might acquire knowledge that is totally precise and fully reliable yet comprehensive. For a belief, construct, or measure to be adequate, two features are needed: 1) *precision*, or the tightness with which it is defined and its intrinsic relationships specified; and 2) *relevance*; it must mean something, in a valid and reliable manner. But the more precisely we define our constructs and formulate their interrelationships, the more likely it becomes that some contradictory datum

179

will emerge that will render our original understanding absurd, ergo less relevant. I had formerly used the term *reliability* for the second variable, but now prefer *relevance* both to allow for multiple contributing inputs and to avoid confusion with the reliability coefficient of statistical measure theory. I stated this inverse relationship between precision and relevance in quasi-mathematical form as $P \times R = C$, where C is a constant whose value remains fixed within a given context of discussion.

The roots of uncertainty, both simple and complex, have in common what I elsewhere term the "A/Not-A Absurdity" (Beahrs, 1982a):

1) A construct (A) is defined as distinct from its negative (not-A) in terms of clear operational variables to which most people can relate.
2) The relevant data are analyzed with intent to clarify what distinguishes A from not-A. In doing so, however,
3) We find irrefutable arguments that what we had originally defined as A is "really" not-A and vice versa, so that the definitions become contradictory and self-defeating even while retaining their clearly specified original meaning.

When this occurs, the construct at hand is said to have lost "relevance"; it no longer applies in a dependable, consistent, reliable, valid or useful manner. Adequacy requires both precision and relevance, but the former can be achieved only at the cost of the latter.

When relevance is impaired, this can occur at two levels: *practical* and *fundamental*. The first can be avoided by changing our understandings or our strategies, while the latter is inherent in the nature of what is. Each can be understood in terms of the logic of the A/Not-A Absurdity.

A pragmatic absurdity arises from the use of arbitrary cutoff points along what is actually a continuum. For example, if state-supported medical health benefits are cut off as soon as a welfare recipient makes over $500 per month, there is a catastrophic loss when a person passes that point that would make him think twice before taking that step. The absurdity is in treating two nearly identical individuals as if they were different, one making $499 and another $501, and associating these with negative motivating consequences. But the absurdity is not logical; it can be circumvented by a continuum that more closely approximates that of actual fact, like the graduated income tax. The latter preserves the greater financial burden on those able to pay, but at no point does the incentive toward greater income become negative.

Two examples will illustrate the A/Not-A Absurdity in everyday living, where it acquires a more fundamental character. A prototype is provided by Donington's (1963) discussion of the limits of perfection in human parenting: The most cruel thing a parent could do to his or her child would be to be *too* perfect. If the parent were beyond reproach in all aspects of quality parenting, the child would have no objective basis against which to rebel and define his own life priorities as a separate person. By being too good, the child is denied one of his most basic needs, and the quality parenting has in itself become an imperfection. But to cut back on the quality of the parenting would be to open the newly introduced flaws to criticism on their own negative merits. The implication of this awareness is that one should generally strive to improve the quality of one's parenting, but that at a certain level any further improvements would paradoxically worsen it. In principle, there should then be a level at which parenting is of optimal quality, beyond which further improvement is *not* possible even in principle. If this could be adequately quantized, it would be approximated by the constant C in the psychic uncertainty relationship.

Another example of where excessive precision turns against itself in psychiatry is the value of the policy manual. Procedural guidelines for handling difficult situations are generally specified in such a manual, to follow accepted professional and medicolegal standards and to provide ground rules to aid the inexperienced clinician. To a point, these are informative as well as protective. But when they pass a point of optimum specificity, it becomes more and more certain that a situation will arise that requires that the guidelines be violated in order to avoid the very type of catastrophe that they were designed to prevent, i.e., they are less reliable or relevant; R (relevance or reliability) has been sacrificed. Often simple human intuition as to what is appropriate will do better in such cases. To avoid such difficulties, attorneys often advise a degree of deliberate looseness in policy manuals, giving leeway to such temporizing concepts as "reasonable" and "medical judgment." Relevance is improved by deliberately sacrificing precision — though to leave all decision-making to "reasonable judgment" would be to obviate the need for professional training, itself an absurdity. An optimal balance between precision and imprecision is clearly needed.

The essential logic of these examples is the A/Not-A Absurdity. Essentially a boundary phenomenon, a simple prototype arises when-

ever we attempt to make a dichotomous choice along what is actually
a continuum in external fact (cf. Figure A.1). The absurdity is revealed
whenever two nearly identical states (D, E) must then be treated as
if they were polar opposites. When the dichotomous choice was unnecessary, the absurdity was practical only. But when the very nature of
our experience *requires* a precise distinction that cannot be reliably
made, it becomes fundamental. The distinction between voluntary and
involuntary action is the example best studied by empirical measure,
and remains the most essential fundamental root of the psychic uncertainty principle.

Uncertainty in mental health *differs* from the quantum uncertainty
principle in the following key respects:

1) The psychic uncertainty constant, C, cannot be given an invariant fixed value determined by experiment, beyond which further
precision of measure is intrinsically impossible. Neither does the uncertainty relationship fit accurately into its simplified linear form, except
in the prototype case of a linear continuum. The relationship $P \times R = C$
is thus not a rigorous mathematical truth, but only a reference to the
inverse nature of the relationship between precision and relevance.
The value of C will differ in one context from another, depending on
the nature and extent of the variables involved. And rather than a
numerical constant, C is more likely to specify a complex function,
but one that remains fixed for the particular context. In mental health,
there will be multiple uncertainty relationships with different mathematical form depending on the component variables at hand.

2) Information that is precluded by the uncertainty principle at one
level may yet be clarified by another variable outside the context, by
viewing the system from a different angle. The value of the limiting
constant C is "fundamental," then, only within a particular specified
context. Going outside or "leaving the field" may have some potential to mitigate its limits. But this new context will then have its own
intrinsic limits, defined by its own inherent uncertainty relationship.
We can escape one particular uncertainty constant by altering our
frame of reference, but we cannot escape the uncertainty principle
itself.

3) That there is a significant component that is truly fundamental
in a more absolute sense can be argued strongly on metapsychological

grounds (below). But there is yet no clear way to delineate the degree
to which the limitation against precision is truly inviolable even in principle, as opposed to being rooted in the correctible inadequacy of our
current knowledge.

4) Some of what gives psychic uncertainty its fundamental quality
are intrinsic factors in the psychological level that are necessarily
beyond measure, such as its essential privacy. The psychic uncertainty
principle therefore remains a philosophical construct that awaits further
mathematical specification and scientific validation, which can never
be complete.

Despite these points of divergence, there are sufficient parallels between the psychic and quantum uncertainty principles to more than
merit an analogy, and only further research data can clarify the degree
to which they truly intersect. The two *parallel* one another in the following ways:

1) Increased precision in one aspect of measure leads to sacrificed
precision in another. In classical physics the entire state of a system
can be specified by only two variables, the position and momentum
of all its constituent parts. But precise measure of position can be
achieved only at the sacrifice of precision in momentum, and vice
versa, so that there is a well quantified limit beyond which further
precision is not possible. This is approached by Planck's constant, h.
The underlying logic follows:

(a) measurement requires a measuring vehicle
(b) the "finest grained" measuring vehicle is the unit of pure energy,
    the photon
(c) high energy of photon alters momentum of what is being meas-
    ured, introducing uncertainty of momentum, Δpx)
(d) high wavelength blurs position of what is being measured, intro-
    ducing uncertainty of position, or Δx)
(e) wavelength and energy of a photon vary *inversely*; $E\lambda \sim h$

Precise specification of momentum can be achieved only at cost of
uncertainty in position, and vice versa. The product of the uncertainties is the overall limit to precision, a numerical constant of the
order of h:

(f) $\Delta p_x \times \Delta x \gtrless h$ (Heisenberg's relationship).

2) A limit against the possibility of tight deterministic knowledge is formally stated in both domains.

3) Both principles argue for a reframing of causal laws, as they apply to their domain, with clear implications for the practice of their associated technologies.

4) In either case, uncertainty follows from two or more reciprocally varying elements, both of which are present at the most fundamental level for the domain in question, and which cannot be reduced to one or the other. For quantum physics, the covariables are the particle aspect vs. the wave aspect of pure energy. For the psychological level in scientific psychiatry, they are the copresence of voluntary and involuntary action or their correlates, conscious and unconscious awareness, in addition to the many untestable intangibles described throughout this book. For the remainder of psychiatry's domain, it is the tension between the need for relatively simple yet precise working principles, pitted against the extraordinary complexity of its actual reality, that prevents such a tight construct from having any universal validity.

These roots will be further clarified in turn. But first there will be a discussion of the historical context, followed by a presentation of the broad logical frame that they share, boundary dilemmas, problems in defining the second variable "reliability" or "relevance," and the mathematical complexities of psychic uncertainty.

THE HISTORICAL CONTEXT

At least a century will generally elapse before philosophical understandings well accepted in the physical sciences are extended to the domain of mental health. Deterministic mechanism, an outgrowth of classical Newtonian physics, actually reached its zenith during the 18th century with the hard determinism of Laplace (Bohm, 1957). If one only knows the "initial conditions" of position and momentum for every element in the universe, one will know with certitude all that has transpired and all that subsequently will be. Although a big "if," such total knowledge is at least "there" in principle, to be ever more closely approached by scientific investigation without finite limit.

Not until the groundbreaking medical advances of vaccination, the germ theory, chemical anesthesia, and radiology did the biological sciences claim their rightful place in this mechanistic universe. Another generation passed before mental health joined the bandwagon at the turn of the century with Freud's essentially hydraulic "psychodynamics" model, explaining much of higher mental processes in terms of often unconscious forces and counterforces (Freud, 1916/1979). Recent advances in psychobiology have held out additional hope for those wishing to understand the mind in mechanistic terms.

As scientific psychiatry has been striving toward its unspoken ideal of classical physics, the underpinnings of this in physics had already crashed in ruins a half-century earlier with the uncertainty principle of Heisenberg (1927), strengthened by Bohr's (1949/1961) argument that deterministic understanding is not possible *even in principle*. The uncertainty principle has changed the very fabric of how physicists look on their "reality," and has already led to such advances as the unification of physics and chemistry under a single theoretical umbrella (Teller, 1980).

There is a similar process occurring in current scientific psychiatry, taking hold most prominently in the current decade. Systems research has only recently shifted the prominent paradigm to a "biopsychosocial model" (Engel, 1980) where a myriad of forces at many levels of organization impinge on the final picture, with more than one being open to therapeutic intervention. Yet the principle of deterministic mechanism, the possibility of increasingly precise formulation without limit to this precision, rarely goes unchallenged as a basic unspoken ideal. It is this ideal that is forbidden by psychic uncertainty. This key principle requires that psychiatry utilize a multilevel systems thinking, a multiaxial diagnostic schema, and a biopsychosocial model where the component levels retain their essentially discrete character.

Groundwork for a psychic uncertainty principle has been laid by many investigators, some of whom will be cited in turn. These contributions are not listed in chronological order but are grouped according to similarities in their concepts. The first six contributions relate to quantum uncertainty, its relationship to causality, and possible intersection with the domain of human living. The next two deal with information theory and the inherent limitation of the information that can be obtained from any system. Another pair addresses the role of the finite and the infinite, and yet another pair moves to the heart of the subjective psychological level. A concluding pair of contributions deals with systems theory at both an objective and cognitive level, with systems thinking being what I have encouraged for the mental health profession throughout this book.

1) *Heisenberg (1927)*: Discovered the classic fundamental limit of reductionistic empirical science, that precision of measure cannot be achieved beyond the order of Planck's constant, h, even in principle. Derivation of this principle is discussed in many popular synopses of modern physics, with an especially lucid summary by Teller (1980). Because of this fundamental limitation, the behavior of subatomic particles can be understood only in terms of a statistical state function, which is altered profoundly by the interaction with the vehicle of measurement. The deterministic laws of classical mechanics remain valid within the limited domain of large-scale objects, and are seen as approximations of the more basic statistical laws of quantum mechanics. The uncertainty principle has paradoxically expanded the scope of science to explain many formerly baffling phenomena, like the periodic table of the chemical elements.

2) *Bohr (1949/1961)*: Considered Heisenberg's uncertainty relationship as only the clearest example of a much broader principle of *complementarity*, which pervades all human knowledge (Folse, 1985). The nature of the human mind allows us to understand something only in classical terms such as space, time, and causality. Where this is not adequate, we need two antithetical points of view, such as the particle/wave duality in matter-energy, that cannot be reduced to one or the other. In biology, Bohr notes the tension between the determinist-reductionistic point of view, and the functional-teleological perspective. In psychology the tension is between seeing one's self as experiencing subject and as observed object. There is a hint of both a subjective as well as objective component to even a physical principle, such as Heisenberg's. Despite Bohr's stature, complementarity has not yet achieved the wide recognition that its author had hoped for.

3) *Sarbin (1944)* also drew a parallel between the uncertainty principle and the domain of psychology: In each case, the act of measurement interferes with what is being measured. Supporting this position, data recently cited by Spanos (1986) illustrate the extent to which

the form of various mental entities is determined by the context in which they are measured, hidden observers being a classic case in point. Rosnow (1983) applies similar reasoning to the domain of social psychology, arguing, as I do, for a "pluralistic" view that accepts "an array of adequate models . . . sensitive to the contexts *and* mechanics of human experience" (p. 334). Nardone (1986) also points out the importance of uncertainty for the clinical reasoning process in general medicine.

4) *Bohm (1957)*: Statistical laws can be approximations of causal laws at a deeper level, as well as vice versa. An uncertainty relationship identical in form to Heisenberg's can be derived for individual smoke particles subjected to the random forces underneath Brownian movement, $\Delta Px \, \Delta X = C$, where C is a function of the temperature. C is not fundamental, since it can be understood in terms of causal forces or "hidden variables" at a deeper level, well within the constraints of quantum uncertainty. Bohm reasons that similar causal variables might underlie Heisenberg's relationship, with the latter being only their common expression. Hidden variable theories have implied slight divergence from standard quantum theory, which has been tested. So far, no hidden variable theory has passed the test.

5) *Comfort (1985)*: Comments on the similarity of the "wave function" used for quantum mechanical systems to "state functions" that could be used to classify different species of higher organisms. He calls upon the life sciences to develop the same type of noncausal thinking that quantum theory has injected into physics. He notes how such basic ways of thinking about reality as time, space, and causality appear to be artifacts of the perceiving mind–brain, rather than an essential feature of physical reality itself. Comfort states: "It has become increasingly hard to characterize the behavior of matter-energy without the insertion of mind as a primitive constituent of the process of definition, which makes the latter circular" (p. 7). He claims that, as in physics, the answer will have to come from outside our current frames of reference.

6) *Zimmerman (1979)*: Questions Bohr's assumption that the mind must perceive reality in classical causal terms, arguing that several centuries ago much of Newtonian physics seemed as "counterintuitive" as quantum phenomena do now. The very nature of how we perceive

reality can and must accommodate to the new discoveries, rather than trying to bend these into an outmoded classical schema.

7) *Szilard (1929)*: Only two years after Heisenberg's principle, noted that any observation actually *removes* information from the context of discussion, that is, we can see something only by ignoring what we do *not* see. As described by Poundstone (1985), *"acquisition of knowledge about one part of the world requires an equal sacrifice of knowledge about other parts"* (p. 76). Information about part of a system can be bought only at the price of sacrificing just as much information about the remainder. Szilard's insight limits the possibility of total deterministic knowledge as irrevocably as Heisenberg's, and to a greater extent, and would remain just as valid were the latter not the case. Poundstone (1985) gives an especially lucid discussion of the logic and implications of Szilard's theorem (pp. 67–77).

Science can be seen as the task of attempting to increase the scope of *useful* information, as opposed to what is less relevant, like the motion of individual gas molecules. In the case of the mind–brain, however, the overall content of relevant information is so vast that to exclude any of it runs the risk that what is excluded can render our explanatory constructs invalid.

8) *Brillouin (1964)*: Clarified the essence of information as order or negative entropy, and using the second law of thermodynamics, showed that any information achieved at one level must be compensated for by an equal or even greater loss in information at another; essentially a demonstration of Szilard's principle from a different angle. In addition, Brillouin points out how *error* is built into many classical mechanical systems in such a manner that it also acquires some fundamental character.

9) *Gödel (1931/1962)*: Demonstrated that any formal system of propositions, logical or mathematical, must remain incomplete; there is a point at which it must prove inconsistent and fall back against itself. Mathematicians are still attempting to unravel the implications of this fundamental constraint, which arises in part from difficulty handling the infinite. Hofstadter (1979) suggests that Gödel's theorem may also follow from the inherent structure of the brain, which, if validated by subsequent experiment, would give it a quality similar to Heisenberg's principle. Hofstadter offers many tantalizing illustrations of "strange

loops" of causality, which come back upon themselves and create logical paradox, illustrating these with examples from the arts.

These paradoxes may emerge from the duality of mind as experiencing subject versus mind as observed object. Hofstadter also points out the *ambiguity* inherent in all language, showing that even rigorous deductive systems like Euclid's proofs contain an essential fuzziness from this very feature alone.

10) *Rucker (1982)*: Presents an especially compelling summary of the many limitations of any finite schema of knowledge in attempting to portray what is actually infinite, without bounds. For any construct, there must be something beyond. The extent to which the complexities of the mind–brain can be looked upon as if infinite must await further study.

To clarify the relationship of a finite construct portraying a greater reality in higher dimensions, I have used the analogy of a two-dimensional photograph of a three-dimensional object like Mt. Rainier (Beahrs, 1982a). Different perspectives can be equally true, but incomplete; the more perspectives we have, the more knowledge of Mt. Rainier is achieved, but no perspective can cover the entire picture.

11) *Bertrand Russell (1948)*: Distinguished between public and private data, noting that the psychological level is of necessity private. He cites the need to distinguish what we know and how we know it, in exploring the limits of our knowledge. And "all the data upon which our inferences should be based are psychological in character; that is to say, they are experiences of single individuals. The apparent publicity of our world is in part delusive and in part inferential; all the raw material of our knowledge consists of mental events in the lives of separate people. In this region, therefore, psychology is supreme" (p. 53). Both the privacy and primacy of the psychological level have subsequently been emphasized by Globus (1973) and myself (Beahrs, 1977a, Essay I).

12) *Stent (1975)*: Claims that the "self" is a fundamental given of human experience and is "transcendental" in that it cannot be dissected into component parts without essential loss of meaning. For this reason, it must escape the grasp of analytic science, *ergo* remain uncertain.

13) *Weiss (1967)*: "Emergent" properties of collective systems cannot be understood in terms of their component parts and therefore

lie beyond reductionistic science alone. Along with von Bertalanffy (1968), Weiss helped develop modern general systems theory. The reductionistic and holistic–systems views are not seen as contradictory but as incomplete in themselves. They are two complementary perspectives equally essential to understanding complex systems, which consist of subsystems, are themselves part of a greater system, and are interdependent with yet other systems. Circular causality is an essential feature of general systems theory.

14) *Koplowitz (1984)*: Extends Piaget's stages of cognitive development beyond formal operations, positing a fourth "systems" stage in which linear causality is replaced by circular causality, and independence of separate entities is replaced by interdependence of systems. There is another subsequent "unitary" stage in which a person recognizes the interconnectedness of nature and appreciates that any entity is essentially a construct of the perceiving organism, with greater or lesser utility as opposed to "truth." Koplowitz further notes that these do not necessarily imply what the essence of objective reality must be, but are simply modes of thinking that become more effective by virtue of the more flexible problem solving they engender.

In such cognitive–developmental terms, the current book can be seen as a call for our profession to develop beyond the mechanistic causality of formal operations to the interdependence of systems thinking and to the relativity of constructs implied by unitary thinking. If these permit a better "fit" with objective reality, then both the styles of thinking as well as their objective correlates are validated.

Several themes occur and recur throughout these discussions. I will include these in three broad categories:

1) *Complex causality*. This encompasses finitude in the face of the infinite, the need for simplicity in the face of the complex, the need for models that are like (n-m)th-dimensional photographs of an n-dimensional reality, hidden variables, and necessary sources of error.
2) *Untestable intangibles of the psychological level*. Foremost among these is the privacy of subjective data and the requirements that all reality be understood within the inherent limits of the human mind–brain. Also at this level are intrinsic ambiguities of language, which in-

clude idiosyncratic word connotations, and the iherent uncertainty in the very definition of free choice, including the value priorities and motivational complexities that contribute to it.

3) *Complementarity between coexisting polar opposites at the psychological level.* This is what I refer to as the "psychic uncertainty principle" proper, that component which most closely parallels the uncertainty principle of Heisenberg. Of these polar opposites, the voluntary/involuntary dichotomy is most basic. Along with its correlate, conscious/unconscious, this is the polarity most open to scientific investigation. Data from the hypnosis research laboratory are the empirical substrate from which I develop psychic uncertainty as fundamental at this level.

BOUNDARY CONTINUA: THE PROTOTYPE

The most simple mathematical prototype of psychic uncertainty arises whenever we need to distinguish a construct (A) from its opposite (Not-A), along what is actually a smooth linear continuum, illustrated in Figure A.1. "Precision" is the tightness of the boundary definitions; it is higher the narrower the boundary or "grey area" that is permitted between A and Not-A. If the boundary is an arbitrary point, then "precision" is considered infinite. But in practice, two virtually identical points on the continuum (D,E) will be treated as if they were opposite, a practical absurdity. If a "grey area" is allowed by deliberately sacrificing precision, like between points m_1 and m_2, only points outside this grey area can be distinguished according to the rules of A/Not-A; since they are necessarily more separate (F,G), the distinction will be more meaningful or "relevant." If precision or P is defined as the reciprocal of the grey area, $C/\Delta x$, so that the word "greater" precision will imply greater numerical value, then relevance or R can simply be the width of the grey area itself, the difference between points before we are permitted to call a point either A nor Not-A. The uncertainty relationship follows as a mathematical tautology. $C/\Delta x \times \Delta x = C$, or $P \times R = C$.

A similar tautology can illustrate the "Adequacy vs. Scope" form of the principle. If criteria are specified for distinguishing A from Not-A so that the definitions will be maximally relevant, such a large grey area will be required that most of the continuum will be excluded,

Figure A.1. The linear continuum

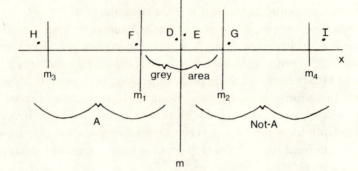

e.g., between points m_3 and m_4. The A/Not-A distinction will be "adequate," or both precisely defined and reliable, but only for a very few cases (like H and I), e.g., at the expense of its scope, or domain (D); $A \times D = C'$. In this limiting case, adequacy corresponds to relevance and scope corresponds to precision.

As specified here, $P \times R = C$ is a rigorous mathematical truth, but only in this limiting prototype case, where practical exigencies require us to make either-or distinctions between A and Not-A when the relevant variable, x, actually varies along a smooth continuum. Here, relevance is simply the measure of the grey area itself, precision its inverse. That they would vary reciprocally is a simple mathematical tautology. What it points toward is the hazard in making arbitrary distinctions that do not reliably correspond to meaningful distinctions in what is actually "out there." This will become fundamental in a meaningful philosophical and scientific sense, only when we examine areas in the domain of mental health *where the intrinsic nature of the variables force us to make these dichotomous distinctions between opposites that can never be separated even in principle* and will thereby be intrinsically unreliable. This is the type of paradox that defines what I intend the psychic uncertainty concept to denote.

THE RELEVANCE CONCEPT

That aspect of precision that is sacrificed by overly tight boundary definitions—what I formerly termed "reliability" and now prefer "relevance"—has been most difficult to define for two reasons: 1) it is intrinsically diffuse—not a unitary variable but a composite of several factors that can lead to the A/Not-A Absurdity; and 2) the terms that common usage would suggest for the second variable, like "reliability" and "validity," have an already well-defined meaning in measure theory, which only partly contributes to the broader "relevance" concept. The following concepts contribute to relevance, to a greater or lesser degree depending upon the situation:

1) *Reliability*. As used in statistical measure theory, "reliability" refers to freedom from error, or from contamination of our construct by extraneous data. The reliability coefficient, r_{tt}, is defined as that component of total variance that is not due to error and that reflects the "true" variance in what is being measured (Kerlinger, 1973). In many situations the word fits the relevance concept quite closely, justifying its original use as the second variable of the uncertainty relationship. This is especially true when validating diagnostic categories in psychiatry, where it is applied to the interrater reliability of the diagnoses—the degree to which different evaluators will concur in the diagnosis, using the same criteria. Williams (1985) has noted the general consensus that multiaxial diagnosis in psychiatry, a deliberate sacrifice of tight boundary definitions, has "contributed substantially . . . to the increased reliability with which they are now diagnosed" (p. 177).

Reliability as the second variable can be quantized whenever A and Not-A can be looked upon as if separate populations, common in actual mental health practice. Figure A.2 depicts a typical curve describing two populations we want to distinguish that overlap. The population "A" is defined mathematically by the area under the f(x) curve, $\int_{-\infty}^{\infty} f(x)$, "Not-A" by the area under a separate curve f'(x), $\int_{-\infty}^{\infty} f'(x)$. The entire population to be evaluated for A vs. Not-A is the sum of the two component curves, $\int_{-\infty}^{\infty} g(x)$ where $g(x) = f(x) + f'(x)$.

The "*probability of misclassification*" (Pmis) is the chance that what is defined as A is really Not-A, or vice versa. If the point of demarcation (m) that arbitrarily defines A from Not-A is taken as the intersection of the two curves, then the absolute Pmis is the portion of the area under the total curve that is contributed by the "wrong" component curve, illustrated by the shaded area, Pmis = $\int_{-\infty}^{m} f'(x) + \int_{m}^{\infty} f(x)$. This is close to a rigorous measure of unreliability.

Figure A.2. Probability of misclassification

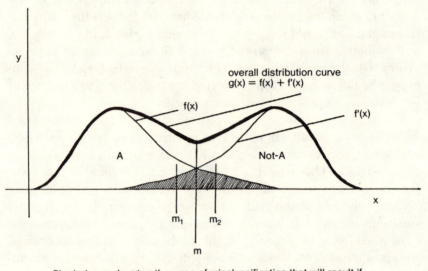

Shaded area denotes the zone of misclassification that will result if
A is arbitrarily distinguished from Not-A by the point m

The difference of m_2-m_1 defines a grey area that excludes much of this zone

The likelihood of misclassification can be lowered significantly by
broadening the demarcation point to include a grey area, within which
the rules of A vs. Not-A do not apply. If A is defined only as $x < m_1$,
and Not-A by $x > m_2$, then the relative probability that what is defined as A is really not-A will be given by $Pmis(A) = \int_{-\infty}^{m_1}[f'(x)/g(x)]$.
The comparable probability of considering as not-A what is really A
is Pmis (Not-A) $= \int_{m_2}^{\infty}[f(x)/g(x)]$.

The larger the grey area, $\Delta x = m_2 - m_1$, the less the probability of
misclassification. This inverse relationship can be defined by $\Delta x \times$
Pmis = C'', the *differential* form of psychic uncertainty. If reliability is
the inverse or reciprocal of Pmis, this translates back to the original
$P \times R = C$, remembering again that the relationship is nonlinear and
complex. The precise mathematical form can be found by the integral
calculus. In general, the larger the gray area permitted between m_1
and m_2, the more the zone of misclassification is removed. Reliability is improved, but at the expense of the A/Not-A distinction's scope.

The word "reliability" is more problematic in cases such as the linear boundary continuum, however, where there is neither measure nor error, but where the inverse relationship between precision and relevance is inherent in the very definition of the situation.

2) *Accuracy* is similar to precision itself, but a precise measure can lose accuracy when it is off target. It implies a consistent systematic error, which is not the intent of the uncertainty principle.

3) *Validity* is another concept used in statistical measure theory, which attempts to get from the measurement situation to what is being measured. A measure is "valid" to the degree that its variance reflects variance in what is being measured. It is that portion of total variance shared by both the measuring instrument and that which it describes. Construct validity is a measure of the degree to which the construct is meaningful, and like reliability, comes close to the second variable of psychic uncertainty. It also correlates highly with low probability of misclassification. A discriminant analysis is often used to determine whether separation of clusters is sufficient to warrant considering them as separate entities, usually requiring that the distance between cluster means (δ) be at least three standard deviations (σ), or $\delta/\sigma \geq 3$ (Snedecor & Cochran, 1967, pp. 414–416).

4) *Common usage terms*. A relevant concept is more or less (a) *dependable*, in that we can count on it; (b) *consistent*, in being replicable; (c) *useful*, in that it predicates constructive techniques that otherwise would be in want of a rationale; (d) *meaningful*, in helping us organize our understanding of the context at hand.

MATHEMATICAL COMPLEXITIES

Many factors make it difficult to put psychic uncertainty into rigorous mathematical formulation, like the one of such value in quantum physics. These factors are:

1) *Uniqueness*. Each context has its own intrinsic uncertainty relationship, depending on the distribution of the variables and the extent to which they fit into separate clusters of A and Not-A as opposed to simply points along a linear continuum. Mathematical complexities inherent in many specific unique systems are:

(a) *nonlinearity*. P and R vary inversely, but in a nonlinear relation-
    ship depending on the shape of the clusters and curves;
(b) C is not a simple constant with a fixed numerical value, but is itself
    a *complex function* constant for any particular context; and
(c) the functions are often highly complex and do not admit well to
    curve-fitting.

Figure A.3 illustrates four different types of distribution. 3a is the
prototype linear continuum of Figure A.1, with no separate construct
validity and the A/Not-A distinction entirely arbitrary. 3b is the opposite and ideal case where A and Not-A are totally separable clusters
with no overlap. In such a case, infinite precision can be achieved with
no sacrifice in reliability; there is no uncertainty relationship in such
cases, or the constant is infinity. 3c depicts a case where there is not
only no cluster separation, like 3a, but A and Not-A merge into a single
cluster with greatest density at the demarcation point. To separate an
A from a Not-A here would be even less reliable than on the linear

Figure A.3. Alternate A/Not-A curves

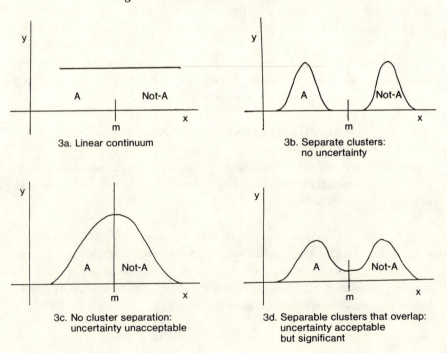

3a. Linear continuum

3b. Separate clusters:
no uncertainty

3c. No cluster separation:
uncertainty unacceptable

3d. Separable clusters that overlap:
uncertainty acceptable
but significant

continuum, reflected in a very low value of C which permits little precision and reliability. 3d represents the type of situation encountered most often in scientific psychiatry, where A and Not-A separate into discrete clusters, but with considerable overlap (already depicted on Figure A.2).

Several factors will help maximize C in the direction of adequacy (high precision with less sacrifice of relevance/reliability); (a) large differential, Δy, or the difference between cluster peaks and their intermediary valley; (b) ratio of $\Delta y max/\Delta y min$; (c) the A/Not-A demarcation point is at a minimum on the curve; and (d) a large absolute slope of the curve on either side of the minimum.

2) *Demarcation point.* This is often hard to define, that is, where to draw the line between A and Not-A. In complex systems there may not be any one "obvious" point, such as the minimum between two clusters, and what is chosen may depend on value priorities.

For example, hypoglycemia vs. nonhypoglycemia appears to follow a linear continuum of minimum blood glucose levels, with the most popular demarcation point for "hypoglycemia" being a level below 50 mg. percent. But as noted elsewhere (Beahrs, 1982b, Appendix I), some argue for a lower cutoff point, others for a higher one, and I have suggested that we deliberately allow a wide grey area within which the distinction is deemed irrelevant. One can also argue that blood glucose is not even the most relevant variable, that the bottom line is whether or not the patient is symptomatic. Yet another criterion would be whether the patient responds to classic treatment with the desired change. These alternate perspectives change the whole frame of reference.

In summary, the uncertainty principle in mental health lacks mathematical rigor not for any intrinsic problem of its own, but because of the various same factors that necessitated the principle in the first place. In short, *the psychic uncertainty principle is subject to its own ravages.*

FUNDAMENTAL ROOTS OF UNCERTAINTY

A. Boundary Dilemmas: The A/Not-A Absurdity

As already discussed, all of the roots of uncertainty in mental health can lead to the A/Not-A Absurdity. These share the common feature of attempting to define constructs with rigorous boundaries when what they denote in objective reality is either more diffuse or more complex. Considered only in this light, the problem is practical and not fundamental. Therefore, this "root" is only a prototype that helps us understand the common expression of the other roots more easily.

The A/Not-A absurdity becomes fundamental only when the nature of our subject matter puts us into a bind: 1) on the one hand, requiring that particular distinctions be made to enhance our ability to conceptualize and act upon our subject matter, and 2) rendering these distinctions essentially unreliable, limiting their relevance. For the limitation to be fundamental rather than practical requires that we demonstrate that the first part of this bind is unavoidable, that is, that the particular distinction is necessary in order to adequately address our subject matter. The reason can be entirely practical, if it is necessarily unavoidable.

B. Complex Causality

This second root of uncertainty depends on the near-infinite complexity of our subject matter and the need for our constructs to be comparatively simple in order to be workable. It is expressed most easily in the "adequacy vs. scope" form, and is that from which the necessity of multiple psychiatric frameworks becomes most clear. The underlying logic follows:

1) Any construct has finite limits.
2) Any construct specifies a certain information content, which excludes an equal or greater amount of information (Brillouin, 1964; Szilard, 1929).
3) The degree of order, information content, or negative entropy is so high that what is excluded retains its relevance, in contrast to nonliving systems. For example, the actions of individual brain cells or patterns of neural activity not specified by a given construct cannot be assumed to be "useless" information like the motion of individual gas molecules which Boyle's law ignores. The amount of useful information contained in the brain is certainly not infinite, but to treat it as if it were might be a useful approximation. In other words, the number of important causal factors is too vast for a single adequate causal formulation.
4) Utility of our constructs depends to a great degree on simplicity (Teller, 1980), or on narrowing their information content.

5) Any theoretical specification about the human mind–brain will necessarily exclude relevant, useful information; therefore, it will be of limited scope.
   (a) A fundamental component of uncertainty arises from the tension between postulate 2 and postulate 3.
   (b) A practical component follows from postulate 4, which is in complementary tension with postulate 3.
6) In either case, causal factors are so extensive and complex that no workable formulation can cover them all; something of relevance must be excluded, thereby limiting the formulation.
7) The more "useful" a construct (what I earlier termed "adequacy"), the more limited its scope; that is, the more information will necessarily be excluded (postulate 2), which will be relevant (3).

Postulate 4 explains the necessity for limited constructs being employed in the first place. Postulate 3 specifies their inability to be reliable. It is the sheer size of the gulf between near infinite complexity of causal factors and the need for simplicity of understanding that imparts a truly fundamental character to this root of uncertainty.

C. Untestable Intangibles of the Psychological Level
   Several inherent features of the psychological level impart a fundamental uncertainty to any attempt at precisely specifying its parameters. These include:

   1) *Privacy and Isolation.*
      (a) *Privacy*
         (i) — Only a specific individual can experience his own existence, which includes his subjective state of being. This is a working assumption of scientific psychiatry which is challenged only by claims of psychics and the occult. Even if partially transgressed at that level, it remains a useful working approximation for modeling the roots of uncertainty. It is simply a way of stating that nobody can read someone else's mind.
         (ii) — We can know the subjective state of another only indirectly, through observation of his behavior and interpretation of this behavior through our own subjective experience.
         (iii) — Knowledge obtained in this way is valid, but conditional

on *trustworthiness* of the behavior, as an honest expression of the subject's internal state, and *validity* of the assumption that one person's subjective states are similar to another's.

(iv) — Both assumptions in (iii) are limited:

a) There is no way to adequately measure the degree that a person presents a behavioral picture which distorts the subject's internal state. Tests currently used to detect malingering in forensic psychiatry are only indirect; they measure consistency of the subject's behavior over time, plus the presence of gross motivating factors in the present. But they remain intrinsically uncertain. For example, one can "trip up" a hypnotic simulator only through aspects of hypnosis that the simulator does not know, like trance logic. The more sophisticated the simulator, the more he can simulate these subtleties as well. Presence of an obvious motivating factor may also argue for malingering, but the very fabric of psychoanalysis is based on the often valid assumption that human motivation does not always follow the rules of rational motivation.

Even more intriguing is the possibility that there might be a component of malingering in all human behavior. A person will always attempt to present only an outward picture that he wants others to have, keeping private material he considers unacceptable. And overt malingering can be a symptom of genuine neurotic illness, although we can also look on a neurotic or narcissistic façade as malingering that has escaped voluntary control and thus become a symptom (cf. Two-and-a-Half, Chapter 7, p. 145). It is likely that a "genuine" and a "malingered" component are both present in most, if not all cases, to a greater or lesser degree. To say that a person is one *or* the other is, therefore, unreliable. When either-or becomes either-and, as in this case, we are now at the fourth fundamental root of psychic uncertainty, which will be presented in turn.

b) Human individuals are both similar to and different from one another. To the degree that people are similar, one can certainly argue that one's own subjective state is probably similar to another's. But people also differ, and in either case the assumption cannot be tested and is intrinsically uncertain. It must remain a philosophical principle.

(b) *Isolation*

(i) — A person can know of something beyond his own self boundaries only indirectly, through the medium of his own subjective state. This is the inverse of the principle of privacy. While science gives the stamp of legitimacy only to what is objective, it is ironic that only the subjective world of one's own experience has any fundamental validity. That is, that is the only place where matter–energy experiences itself (Beahrs, 1977a, Essay 1).

(ii) — Knowledge of external reality can be validated only indirectly: by consensus with other individuals, which includes the historical dialect of dominating argument, and by consistency of measure. The latter is the cornerstone of all science. In a sense, the domain of science may be defined by the extent to which these criteria apply. Much, if not most, of another person's subjective experience necessarily lies beyond these bounds.

(iii) — Many features that we perceive as fundamental to the nature of reality are artifacts of the structure of the mind–brain. For exmple, such basic concepts as time, space, and causality have little meaning for describing external reality at the most fundamental level, as quantum physicists increasingly realize. They are better seen as artifacts of the perceiving organism, "constructs" by which we organize our experience of reality. Like all constructs, they have limited scope and are constrained by the information that is excluded from their definitions.

(iv) — Some objective reality is assumed to exist, independently of the observing individual. Required for science to have any meaning, this nonetheless remains an assumption.

(v) — All human knowledge involves a complementary interaction between an objective reality and a perceiving organism, with the form of the knowledge determined by both and adequately determined by neither.

Heisenberg's uncertainty principle in quantum physics represents the most objective component of uncertainty, having arisen unexpectedly from rigorous experiment, validated again and again by both consensus and consistency of measure, and amenable to precise quantification. Yet the very form in which it is stated implies the concepts of time and causality, which quantum physicists acknowledge are partly artifacts of the perceiving organism. Therefore, a psychological component contributes to even this most objective level. Heisenberg's principle can best be seen as the extreme limit of what a human individual can understand about external reality in the causal terms in which he thinks; the limit thus follows from both "what is" in objective reality and the nature of the perceiving mind–brain.

2) *Ambiguity of Language*.

(a) Language is inherently imprecise, with multiple levels of meaning, implication, and connotation always present. This is increasingly well recognized in the scientific study of linguistics, semantics and syntactics.
(b) Individuals vary profoundly in these levels of implication.
(c) All scientific knowledge requires language for its formulation, understanding, and communication.
(d) Ambiguity of language places a fundamental constraint against scientific precision, due to all factors above.

3) *Indeterminacy of Free Choice*.

(a) Free choice is inherently indeterministic, at least in the sense of being *self*-determined (Beahrs, 1977a, Essay III).
(b) "Freedom" increases to the extent that the choosing self has a greater number of alternatives from which it can choose (Beahrs, 1977a, Essay III).
(c) The nature of a particular choice is often *binary*, requiring a decision "for" or "against" something, excluding alternatives that would be equally valid.
(d) To the extent that free choice is taken as a basic "given," uncertainty is inherent in the context.
(e) The psychological level is that level at which free choice is basic, by definition (see Chapter 3).
(f) Uncertainty is therefore inherent in the defining characteristics of the psychological level.

The issue of free will vs. determinism remains an age–old philosophical dilemma, which is still argued as strongly as ever. My own position remains a "compatibilist" one, that free choice may require a certain deterministic order to even become possible (Beahrs, 1977a, Essay III, Ch. 3). The relatively large size of the human organism may be needed in order for freedom *not* to be influenced too much by quantum fluctuations. "Freedom" is relevant only at a particular level, which does not exclude investigation of its underlying mechanisms at deeper levels. Hence, I would not argue free choice as a fundamental root of uncertainty, except at the level where it is given primacy by definition. At this level it is a tautology.

The next section presents empirical research data, which suggest that free choice is not unitary but occurs at many simultaneous co-conscious levels. Uncertainty becomes fundamental when we need to distinguish between whether or not an awareness was "conscious" or an action "voluntary," relative to a whole person, when in actual fact it both was and was not. Inseparability of voluntary and involuntary action, and conscious and unconscious awareness, is where uncertainty in specifying consciousness and volition becomes fundamental. This is the root of psychic uncertainty closest in forms to Heisenberg's principle, but it is not to be misconstrued as deriving from it. It emerges from its own independent empirical data and confirmation.

D. Complementarity of Polar Opposites at the Psychological Level

The empirical data supporting co-consciousness are presented in depth elsewhere (Beahrs, 1982b, Appendix I; Beahrs, 1983), as well as being summarized in Chapter 5 of this book. This discussion outlines the core logic, as follows:

1) The basic units of the psychological level are conscious awareness and voluntary action. This is true, by definition of the psychological level. Consciousness and volition imply an experiencing "self," which is not divisible without intrinsic loss of meaning (Stent, 1975). However, the definition does not require that they be unitary; instead, it requires that if we postulate component parts of a self, staying at the psychological level, these parts must also have their own relative sense of consciousness and volition. The extent to which this is actually the case awaits extensive experimental scrutiny, which has been accomplished to date only within the hypnosis laboratory.

2) Precise distinctions between conscious/unconscious awareness or voluntary/involuntary action *must be made*, by scientific psychiatry as well as common language. Common usage, social action, as well as psychiatric classification, all require these distinctions. They are inherent in the following areas of discourse:

(a) *Responsibility*: If an individual kills another, for example, the crime with which he is charged will vary profoundly according to the degree of voluntariness or *mens rea* presumed (e.g., first-degree murder, manslaughter, negligent homicide, or simple accident, in decreasing order). The insanity defense is only an awkward legal formalization of this awareness.

(b) *Everyday experience*: There is a profound subjective difference between purposely lifting one's hand and experiencing it as "just happening," as in a hand levitation; the experience is often either-or in character. Similarly, how we judge others depends on our assessment of whether another "really meant" to do what he did. Many essential subtleties that determine our behavior depend on our assessment of this level (e.g., whether to confront another directly or indirectly, and matters of tact and timing).

(c) *Scientific psychiatry*: Distinguishing real vs. malingered illness.

3) Voluntary action cannot be separated from involuntary action, or conscious from unconscious awareness, *even in principle*, at least relative to a whole person. This postulate is argued through the parallel dichotomy of hypnosis vs. nonhypnosis, which contains volition vs. nonvolition as an essential defining feature (see Chapter 5). The argument is based on empirical data summarized as follows:

(a) Hypnosis cannot be precisely distinguished from nonhypnosis without logical absurdity. This is a summary of voluminous research collectively termed the "skeptical" and was my original prototypic scientific illustration of the A/Not-A Absurdity (Beahrs, 1982b, Appendix I).

(b) What applies to hypnosis must to some degree apply to nonhypnosis as well, and vice versa.

(c) Co-conscious mental units or "hidden observers" are an essential feature of normal hypnosis. This is a summary of more voluminous "neodissociation" research (Hilgard, 1977), elaborated upon by Watkins and Watkins' (1979a) discovery of multiple hidden observers coexisting in the same normal subjects.

(d) Co-consciousness is an important feature of normal waking human experience. This is a conclusion from postulates 3b–c and is thus a logical synthesis of the data arising from the skeptical and neodissociation research. To be fully scientific, the conclusion as well as its premises must be tested. Preliminary validation comes from the psychiatric consulting room:

(i) — Hidden ego states often emerge when called for.

(ii) — Interpretation of some "unconscious" element often leads to reactions like relief, tension, or show of understanding, which imply that at some level the individual knew the content of the interpretation all along and yet did not know it overtly until confronted.

(iii) — Response to paradoxical directives often has a sense of immediacy that is hard to attribute to nonsentient mechanism. In other words, the assumption of co-consciousness is eminently testable, and what is well known to work in the consulting room provides preliminary empirical validation of relevance of the co-consciousness concept. Much research is needed to define its limits of relevance.

(e) Relative to a single human individual, it is impossible to separate hypnosis from nonhypnosis, or voluntary from involuntary action, because it is *both at once*, depending on from what perspective the situation is viewed.

(f) There is no way to determine that one perspective is more valid than another.

4) The uncertainty relationship is fundamental at the psychological level. This postulate is a necessary conclusion from postulates 2 and 3. The third postulate necessitates the blurred boundary between overall voluntariness and involuntariness, due to its inherent multiplicity. That the uncertainty is fundamental, not just practical, follows from the second postulate, which requires that we make the distinctions in the first place.

5) The nature and role of the "autonomous I" will clarify the parameters of psychic uncertainty and await further research. Uncertainty follows from our inability to determine from what reference point to judge whether or not something was conscious or voluntary. If one reference point can ever be designated as more valid than another, in a way that is consistently testable and open to scientific consensus, then we could designate whether or not something was conscious, voluntary, or hypnotic, relative to that reference point. Whether or not there can be such a point is not known, however. Hilgard (1977) has summarized two alternative viewpoints about the executive function:

(a) Overall selfhood, or the executive function, could arise from a competing hierarchy of lesser drives or ego states, like government in an ideal democracy; or

(b) Executive function might follow from a separate agency that we simply do not yet know of.

(c) If (a), then uncertainty remains fundamental for reasons already discussed.

(d) If (b), a portion of its fundamental quality may be relieved, but the practical component of uncertainty will remain in most cases. This also must await more data. Where self proper is distinct and reliable, uncertainty will be minimal; where not, it will still reign. As everywhere else, it will vary from situation to situation.

(e) Even if a separate agency were definable, some uncertainty remains in the fact that "self proper" identifies with more than one of its component ego states at the same time.

In the example of the driver who was driving automatically while actively planning the next week with his wife (see Chapter 5, p. 94), the "driver" was considered hypnotized but the life planner not. But self proper identified with each and thus to some degree transcended the separate states. Relative to even self proper, then, we cannot reliably say the individual is either hypnotized or not. At this level, the fundamental quality is retained.

IMPLICATIONS OF UNCERTAINTY IN MENTAL HEALTH

This entire book has illustrated the theoretical and practical implications of uncertainty at many levels of scientific psychiatry. Here is a brief summary list, again in outline form.

A. Allowing Grey Areas

Reliability and/or relevance of our constructs is often enhanced by deliberate imprecision by allowing a grey area between A and Not-A where the rules of A/Not-A are acknowledged not to apply. Examples are:

1) graduated income tax is better than single arbitrary cutoff points;
2) liberal use of the word "atypical" in DSM-III improves the manual's utility;

3) multiaxial diagnosis improves the reliability of psychiatric diagnosis

B. *Either-Or Questions Reframed*
   Either-*and* replaces either-or.

1) to what degree?
2) at what level?
3) when different levels conflict, what level takes precedence over others, for the decision at hand?

C. *Concepts of Causality Redefined*
   1) "Truth" often replaced by "relevance" and "utility."
   2) "Cause" often replaced by "focal point."
   3) Absolute validation often replaced by "legitimacy."
   4) Certainty often replaced by the "presumption" in favor of the status quo, or the socially legitimate.
      (a) Moral presumption.
      (b) Factual presumption.
      (c) Therapeutic presumption.

D. *Unification Replaced by Integration or Coordination*
   1) Conductor-orchestra analogy.
      (a) Ego states comprising a single human self.
      (b) Multiple psychiatric systems or modalities required.
      (c) Executive function needed.
         (i) — awaits research.
         (ii) — determination is currently pragmatic.
   2) Multiaxial diagnosis more reliable.
   3) Need for Differential Therapeutic Index.
      (a) Impossible to unify psychiatry into single adequate system.
      (b) Multiple systems or modalities needed.
      (c) Executive system needed to coordinate sub-systems; Axis VI proposed.

CONCLUDING ILLUSTRATIONS: LEAVING THE FIELD

One unique feature of uncertainty in the domain of mental health is an ability to "leave the field" or to shift our theoretical and practiced frame of reference when needed, a point emphasized throughout this book. Two earlier case examples will provide a concluding illustration of two aspects of this process; the need for multiple models and the primacy of value priorities.

Mrs. R, the case prototype described in the Introduction and Chapter 8, presented with a history of recurrent psychosis. As the patient had an intact cognitive mental status, the traditional differential diagnosis was between schizophrenia and bipolar disorder. But this dichotomy was not "relevant" for her; neither alternative provided understanding or effective treatment. It was necessary to shift gears and find an alternative frame of reference — in short, to leave the field. Figure A.4 depicts the process. The bold lines, 4a, depict the schizophrenic/bipolar distinction. If we denote Mrs. R's psychosis by point R on the diagram, it clearly fits into a zone of nonrelevance. But to think of her in terms of a superimposed dichotomy, hypnosis/nonhyp-

Figure A.4. Leaving the field

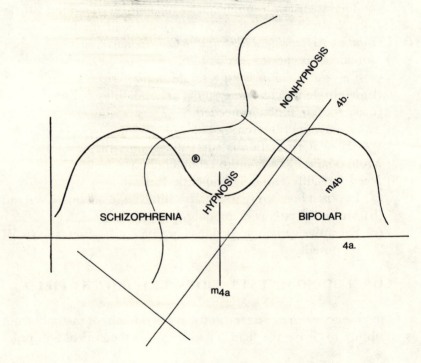

nosis (lighter lines, 4b), proved more fruitful and led to successful resolution of the problem. We can think of the domain of psychiatry as encompassing many such superimposed A/Not-A curves. Each is inherently uncertain; the trick is finding the one for which the uncertainty is least problematic in a particular case.

Coffee Addict (Chapter 2) represented a patient whose psychodynamics were clear and obvious, and appeared to warrant long-term psychoanalytic treatment whose course seemed predictable. Only when massive caffeine abuse was identified did an alternative treatment appear, to discontinue coffee, so superior in time and cost efficiency that the analytic formulation lost relevance. This would render psychoanalysis inappropriate, by clear criteria upon which most psychiatrists would agree.

But a devil's advocate can raise an intriguing counterargument: Suppose that the coffee abuse were missed, as happens all too often in clinical practice, and that the patient had been psychoanalyzed. It is possible that eventually he might have reaped the positive benefits that psychoanalytic theory had predicted, even with the ongoing caffeine abuse. Although the massive expenditure in time, cost, and emotional stress could easily have been avoided, it is at least possible that the patient would now be a much stronger person than otherwise, and that this strength might benefit him in ways that we can only speculate upon.

The point of this concluding illustration is to emphasize that the type of choice on which differential therapeutics so often rest cannot be reduced to only scientific principles, but must ultimately depend on the value priorities of the individuals involved and the society to which they contribute. This is the limit of scientific psychiatry.

Bibliography

Aiken, R. (1981). *Multidimensional man*. New York: Penguin.

Allison, R. B. (1974). A new treatment approach for multiple personalities. *American Journal of Clinical Hypnosis, 17,* 15–32.

Allison, R. B. (1978). A rational psychotherapy plan for multiplicity. *Svensk Tidskrift for Hypnos,* No. 3–4, 9–16.

Allison, R. B. & Schwarz, T. (1980). *Minds in many pieces*. New York: Rawson, Wade.

American Psychiatric Association. (1973). *Megavitamin and orthomolecular therapy in psychiatry*. Task Force, Reprint #7. Washington, DC: Author.

American Psychiatric Association. (1980). *Diagnostic and statistical manual of mental disorders* (3rd ed.). Washington, DC: Author.

American Psychiatric Association. (1984, May). Does psychodynamic theory have little relevance to comtemporary psychiatric care? Unpublished debate, T. B. Karasu, (Moderator), Annual meeting, Los Angeles.

Andreason, N. C., Endicott, J., Spitzer, R. L., & Winokur, G. (1977). The family history method using diagnostic criteria. *Archives of General Psychiatry, 34,* 1229–1235.

Anthony, D., Dippe, S., Hofeldt, F., Daris, J., & Forsham, P. (1973). Personality disorder and reactive hypoglycemia: A quantitative study. *Diabetes, 22,* 664.

Arieti, S. (1976). *Creativity, the magic synthesis*. New York: Basic Books.

Assagioli, R. (1973). *The act of will*. New York: Penguin.

Atkinson, R. & Swizegood, T. (1983). Moral pain and guilt in Vietnam veterans. Unpublished paper, Psychiatric Grand Rounds, Portland, Oregon VA Medical Center.

Bach, G. R. & Torbet, L. (1983). *The inner enemy: How to fight fair with yourself*. New York: William Morrow & Co.

Bakker, C. B. & Bakker-Rabdau, M. K. (1973). *No trespassing! Explorations in human territoriality*. San Francisco: Chandler & Sharp.

Baldessarini, R. (1985). *Chemotherapy in psychiatry*. (2nd ed.). Cambridge, MA: Harvard University Press.

Bandler, B. & Grinder, J. (1975). *The structure of magic, Vols. I & II*. Palo Alto, CA: Science & Behavior Books.

Barber, T. X. (1972). An alternative paradigm. In E. Fromm & R. E. Shor (Eds.), *Hypnosis: Research developments and perspectives* (pp. 115–182). Chicago/New York: Aldine-Atherton.

Barnard, C. I. (1938). *The functions of the executive*. Cambridge, MA: Harvard University Press.

Barnes, G. (1977). *Transactional analysis after Eric Berne: Teaching and practices of three TA schools*. New York: Harper & Row.

Beahrs, J. O. (1971). The hypnotic psychotherapy of Milton H. Erickson. *American Journal of Clinical Hypnosis, 14,* 73–90.

Beahrs, J. O. (1977a). *That which is: An inquiry into the nature of energy, ethics and mental health*. Portland, OR: Integrated Arts, Inc.*

---

*For information about how to obtain copies of *That Which Is* and unpublished material, contact the author at 3318 N.E. Hancock St., Portland, OR 97212.

Beahrs, J. O. (1977b). Integrating Erickson's approach. *American Journal of Clinical Hypnosis, 20*, 55–68.

Beahrs, J. O. (1980). Cure: An opportunity for yes-butting. *Transactional Analysis Journal, 10*, 131–132.

Beahrs, J. O. (1982a). Understanding Erickson's approach. In J. K. Zeig (Ed.), *Ericksonian approaches to hypnosis and psychotherapy.* New York: Brunner/Mazel.

Beahrs, J. O. (1982b). *Unity and multiplicity: Multilevel consciousness of self in hypnosis, psychiatric disorder and mental health.* New York: Brunner/Mazel.

Beahrs, J. O. (1983). Co-consciousness: A common denominator in hypnosis, multiple personality and normalcy. *The American Journal of Clinical Hypnosis, 26,* 100–113.

Beahrs, J. O. & Humiston, K. E. (1974). Dynamics of experiential therapy. *American Journal of Clinical Hypnosis, 17,* 1–14.

Bebbington, P. (1980). Causal models and logical inference in epidemiological psychiatry. *British Journal of Psychiatry, 137,* 317–325.

Beck, A. T. (1976). *Cognitive therapy and the emotional disorders.* New York: International Universities Press.

Beck, A. T. & Emery, G. (1985). *Anxiety disorders and phobias: A cognitive perspective.* New York: Basic Books.

Bell, I. R. (1982). *Clinical ecology: A new medical approach to environmental illness.* Bolinas, CA: Commonwealth Research Institute.

Bellak, L. (1970). *The porcupine dilemma: Reflections on the human condition.* New York: Citadel Press.

Bellak, L. & Small, L. (1978). *Emergency psychotherapy and brief psychotherapy* (2nd ed.). New York: Grune & Stratton.

Benson, H. & Klipper, M. (1976). *The relaxation response.* New York: Avon.

Berne, E. (1961). *Transactional analysis in psychotherapy.* New York: Grove Press.

Berne, E. (1964). *Games people play.* New York: Grove Press.

Berne, E. (1966). *Principles of group treatment.* New York: Oxford University Press.

Berne, E. (1972). *What do you say after you say hello?* New York: Grove Press.

Bernheim, H. (1947). *Suggestive therapeutics.* New York: London Book Co. (Original work published 1890)

Beutler, L. E. (1979). Toward specific psychological therapies for specific conditions. *Journal of Consulting and Clinical Psychology, 47,* 882–897.

Bleuler, E. (1952). *Dementia praecox, or the group of schizophrenias.* New York: International Universities Press. (Original work published 1911)

Bliss, E. L. (1980). Multiple personalities: A report of 14 cases with implications for schizophrenia and hysteria. *Archives of General Psychiatry, 37,* 1338–1397.

Bohm, D. (1957). *Causality and chance in modern physics.* Philadelphia: University of Pennsylvania Press.

Bohm, D. (1971). Quantum theory as an indication of a new order in physics. Part A. The development of new orders as shown through the history of physics. *Foundations of Physics, 1,* 359–381.

Bohm, D. (1980). *Wholeness and the implicate order.* London: Routledge & Kegan-Paul.

Bohr, N. (1961). *Atomic physics and human knowledge.* New York: Science Editions, Inc. (Original work published 1949)

Boyer, T. H. (1985). The classical vacuum. *Scientific American, 253*(2), 70–78.

Braun, B. G. (1983). Psychophysiologic phenomena in multiple personality and hypnosis. *The American Journal of Clinical Hypnosis, 26*(2), 124–137.

Braun, B. G. (1984). Towards a theory of multiple personality and other dissociative phenomena. In B. G. Braun (Ed.), Multiple personality. *Psychiatric Clinics of North America, 7*(1), 171–193.

Breuer, J. & Freud, S. (1955). *Studies on hysteria.* New York: Basic Books. (Original work published 1895)

Brill, E. H. (1979). *The Christian moral vision* (p. 43). New York: The Seabury Press.

Brillouin, L. (1964). *Scientific uncertainty and information.* New York/London: Academic Press.

Brodsky, C. M. (1983). Allergic to everything: A medical subculture. *Psychosomatics, 24,* 731–742.

Campbell, R. J. (1981). *Psychiatric dictionary* (5th ed.). New York/Oxford: Oxford University Press.

Caputo, P. (1977). *A rumor of war.* New York: Random House.

Carnegie, D. (1936). *How to win friends and influence people.* New York: Simon & Schuster.

Comfort, A. (1985). On physic and biology: Getting our act together. *Perspectives in Biology and Medicine, 29,* 1–9.

Dickey, L. D. (Ed.). (1976). *Clinical ecology,* Springfield, IL: CC Thomas.

Dollard, J. & Miller, N. (1950). *Personality and psychotherapy.* New York: McGraw-Hill.

Donington, R. (1963). *Wagner's "Ring" and its symbols.* London: Faber & Faber.

Edelstien, M. G. (1981). *Trauma, trance, and transformation: A clinical guide to hypnotherapy.* New York: Brunner/Mazel.

Edmonston, W. E. (1972). Relaxation as an hypnotic experimental control in hypnosis. *American Journal of Clinical Hypnosis, 14,* 218–229.

Ehrenwald, J. (1978). *The esp experience: A psychiatric validation.* New York: Basic Books.

Einstein, A. (1936). Physics and reality. *Journal of the Franklin Institute, 221.*

Ellis, A. (1962). *Reason and emotion in psychotherapy.* Secaucus, NJ: Lyle Stewart.

Engel, G. L. (1962). *Psychological development in health and disease.* Philadelphia: Saunders.

Engel, G. L. (1980). The clinical application of the biopsychosocial model. *The American Journal of Psychiatry, 137,* 535–544.

English, F. (1977). What shall I do tomorrow?: Reconceptualizing transactional analysis. In G. Barnes (Ed.), *Transactional analysis after Eric Berne: Teachings and practices of three TA schools* (pp. 287–347). New York: Harper & Row.

Erickson, M. H. (1983). *Healing in hypnosis.* New York: Irvington.

Erickson, M. H. & Rossi, E. L. (1979). *Hypnotherapy: An exploratory casebook.* New York: Irvington.

Eysenck, H. J. (1980). A unified theory of psychotherapy, behavior therapy, and spontaneous remission. *Z. Psycho. Bd., 188.*

Feighner, J. P., Robins, E., Guze, S. B., Woodruff, R. A., Winokur, G., & Munoz, R. (1972). Diagnostic criteria for use in psychiatric research. *Archives of General Psychiatry, 26,* 57–63.

Feigl, H. (1967). *The mental and the physical.* Minneapolis: University of Minneapolis Press.

Feynman, R. P., Leighton, R. B. & Sands, M. (1963). *The Feynman lectures on physics.* Menlo Park, CA: Addison-Wesley.

First, H. G. (1980). Anatomy of resistance to the emergent paradigm: Orthomolecular medicine. *Journal of Orthomolecular Psychiatry, 9*, 253–262.

Flavell, J. (1963). *The developmental psychology of Jean Piaget*. New York: Van Nostrand.

Folse, H. J. (1985). *The philosophy of Neils Bohr: The framework of complementarity*. Amsterdam: North Holland.

Fowler, J. E., Budzynski, J. H., & Vandenbergh, R. L. (1976). Effects of an EEG biofeedback relaxation program on the control of diabetes: A case study. *Biofeedback and Self-Regulation, 1*, 105–111.

Frances, A. & Clarkin, J. F. (1981). No treatment as the prescription of choice. *Archives of General Psychiatry, 38*, 542–545.

Frances, A., Clarkin, J. F., & Perry, S. (1984a). *Differential therapeutics in psychiatry: The art and science of treatment selection*. New York: Brunner/Mazel.

Frances, A., Clarkin, J. F., & Perry, S. (1984b). DSM-III and family therapy. *American Journal of Psychiatry, 141*, 406–409.

Frank, J. O. (1973). *Persuasion and healing: A comparative study of psychotherapy*. Baltimore: Johns Hopkins University Press.

Frank, J. D. (1984). Nuclear death: An unprecedented challenge to psychiatry and religion. *The American Journal of Psychiatry, 141*(11), 1343.

Frankel, F. H. (1976). *Hypnosis: Trance as a coping mechanism*. New York/London: Plenum Medical Book Co.

Frankl. V. E. (1978). *The unheard cry for meaning: Psychotherapy and humanism*. New York: Simon & Schuster.

Fredericks, C. (1976). *Psychonutrition*. New York: Grosset & Dunlap.

Freud, S. (1933). *New introductory lectures on psychoanalysis* (J. Strachey, ed. & trans.). New York: W. W. Norton.

Freud, S. (1961). *Civilization and its discontents* (J. Strachey, ed. & trans.). New York: W. W. Norton. (Original work published 1930)

Freud, S. (1971). *Psychopathology of everyday life* (J. Strachey, ed., A. Tyson, trans.). New York: W. W. Norton. (Original work published 1904)

Freud, S. (1975). *Beyond the pleasure principle* (J. Strachey, ed. & trans.). New York: W. W. Norton (Original work published 1920)

Freud, S. (1979). *Introductory lectures on psychoanalysis* (J. Strachey, trans.). New York: Liveright. (Original work published 1916)

Freud, S. (1979). *Group psychology and the analysis of the ego* (J. Strachey, ed. & trans.). New York: W. W. Norton. (Original work published 1921)

Freud, S. (1980). *Interpretation of dreams* (J. Strachey, ed.). New York: Avon. (Original work published 1900)

Fromm, E. (1956). *The art of loving*. New York: Harper & Bros.

Fromm, E. (1973). *The anatomy of human destructiveness*. New York: Holt, Rhinehart & Winston.

Galanter, M. (1982). Charismatic religious sects and psychiatry: An overview. *American Journal of Psychiatry, 139*, 12.

Gallwey, W. T. (1976). *Inner tennis: Playing the game*. New York: Random House.

Gedo, J. E. & Goldberg, A. (1973). *Models of the mind: A psychoanalytic theory*. Chicago: The University of Chicago Press.

Gill, M. M. & Brenman, M. (1959). *Hypnosis and related states: Psychoanalytic studies in regression*. New York: International Universities Press.

Globus, G. G. (1973). Consciousness and brain. *Archives of General Psychiatry, 29*, 153–176.

Gödel, K. (1962). *On formally undecidable propositions*. New York: Basic Books (Original work published 1931)

Goulding, M. M. & Goulding, R. L. (1979). *Changing lives through redecision therapy*. New York: Brunner/Mazel.

Green, H. (1964). *I never promised you a rose garden*. New York: Holt, Rhinehart & Winston.

Greenspan, S. I. & Sharfstein, S. S. (1981). Efficacy of psychotherapy. *Archives of General Psychiatry, 38*, 1213-1219.

Grieco, M. H. (1982). Controversial practices in allergy. *Journal of the American Medical Association, 247*, 3106-3111.

Grinker, R. R., Sr. (1975). The relevance of general systems theory to psychiatry. In S. Arieti (Ed.), *American handbook of psychiatry* (Vol. VI, pp. 251-271). New York: Basic Books.

Groder, M. (1977). Groder's 5 OK Diagrams. In G. Barnes (Ed.), *Transactional analysis after Eric Berne: Teachings and practices of three TA schools*. New York: Harper & Row.

Gruenewald, D. (1977). Multiple personality and splitting phenomena: A reconceptualization. *Journal of Nervous and Mental Diseases, 164*, 385.

Haley, J. (1963). *Strategies of Psychotherapy*. New York: Grune & Stratton.

Haley, J. (1971). *Uncommon therapy: The psychiatric techniques of Milton H. Erickson, M.D.*. New York: Norton.

Haley, J. (1978). *Problem solving therapy*. San Francisco: Jossey-Bass.

Harriman, P. L. (1943). A new approach to multiple personalities. *American Journal of Orthopsychiatry, 13*, 636.

Harris, S. (1936). The diagnosis and treatment of hyperinsulinism. *Annals of Internal Medicine, 10*, 514-533.

Haykin, M. D. (1980). Type casting: The influence of early childhood experience upon the structure of the Child ego state. *Transactional Analysis Journal, 10*, 354-364.

Hebb, D. O. (1949). *Organization of Behavior*. New York: Wiley.

Heisenberg, W. (1927). Über den anschaulichen inhalt der quantentheoretischen kinematik und mechanik. *Zeitschrift fur Physik, 43*, 172-198.

Hilgard, E. R. (1968). *The experience of hypnosis: A shorter version of hypnotic susceptibility*. New York: Harcourt, Brace & World.

Hilgard, E. R. (1977). *Divided consciousness: Multiple controls in human thought and action*. New York: John Wiley & Sons.

Hilgard, E. R. & Hilgard, J. R. (1975). *Hypnosis in the relief of pain*. Los Altos, CA: William Kaufman.

Hilgard, J. R. (1970). *Personality and hypnosis: A study of imaginative involvement*. Chicago: University of Chicago Press.

Hofeldt, F. D., Adler, R. A., & Herman, R. H. (1975). Postprandial hypoglycemia, fact or fiction? *Journal of the American Medical Association, 233*, 1309.

Hoffer, J. (1974). Orthomolecular therapy: An examination of the issues. Regina, Saskatchewan, Canada, Canadian Schizophrenia Foundation.

Hofstadter, D. R. (1979). *Gödel, Escher, Bach: An eternal golden braid*. New York: Basic Books.

Holton, G. (1970). The roots of complementarity. *Daedalus, 99*, 1015-1055.

Horowitz, M. J. (1980). Pathological grief and the activation of latent self-images. *American Journal of Psychiatry, 137*, 1157-1162.

Jackson, D. D. (1957). The question of family homeostasis. *Psychiatric Quarterly Supplement, (31)*, 79-90.

Jahn, D. L. & Lichstein, K. L. (1980). The resistive client: A neglected phenomenon in behavior therapy. *Behavior Modification, 4*, 303-320.

James, M. (1979). *Marriage is for loving*. Reading, MA: Addison-Wesley.

James, M. & Jongeword, D. (1971). *Born to win: Transactional analysis with Gestalt experiments.* Reading, MA: Addison-Wesley.

James, W. (1890). *Principles of psychology.* New York: Dover.

James, W. (1961). *The varieties of religious experience.* New York: Macmillan. (Original work published 1902)

Jung, C. G. (1961). *Memories, dreams, and reflections.* New York: Random House.

Jung, C. G. (1964). *Man and his symbols.* London: Aldus Books.

Kampman, R. (1976). Hypnotically induced multiple personality: An experimental study. *International Journal of Clinical and Experimental Hypnosis, 24,* 215–227.

Karasu, T. B. (1979). Toward unification of psychotherapies: A complementary model. *American Journal of Psychotherapy, 33,* 555–563.

Karasu, T. B. (1982). Psychotherapy and pharmacotherapy: Toward an integrative model. *American Journal of Psychiatry, 139,* 1102–1113.

Karasu, T. B. (1984). *The psychiatric therapies.* Washington, DC: American Psychiatric Association.

Karasu, T. B. & Skodel, A. A. (1980). VIth axis for DSM-III: Psychodynamic evaluation. *American Journal of Psychiatry, 137,* 607–610.

Karpman, S. B. (1968). Fairy tales and script drama analysis. *Transactional Analysis Bulletin, 7.* 39–43.

Kaslow, F. & Sussman, M. B. (1982). *Cults and the family.* New York: Haworth Press.

Kazdin, A. E. & Hersen, M. (1980). The current status of behavior therapy. *Behavior Modification, 4,* 283–302.

Kerlinger, F. N. (1973). *Foundations of behavioral research.* New York: Holt, Rinehart & Winston.

Kernberg. O. (1975). *Borderline conditions and pathological narcissism.* New York: Jason Aronson.

Kilmann, P. R., Scoveru, A. W., & Moreault, D. (1979). Factors in the patient-therapist interaction and outcome: A review of the literature. *Comprehensive Psychiatry, 20,* 132–146.

Klerman, G. L., Weissman, M. M., Rounsaville, B. J. & Chevron, E. S. (1984). *Interpersonal psychotherapy of depression.* New York: Basic Books.

Kline, M. V. (1972). Freud and hypnosis: A re-evaluation. *Journal of Clinical and Experimental Hypnosis, 20*(4), 252–263.

Kluft, R. P. (1982). Varieties of hypnotic interventions in the treatment of multiple personality. *American Journal of Clinical Hypnosis, 24,* 230–240.

Kohut, H. (1966). Forms and transformations of narcissism. *Journal of the American Psychoanalytic Association, 14,* 243–272.

Kohut, H. (1971). *The analysis of the self.* New York: International Universities Press.

Kohut, H. (1977). *The restoration of the self.* New York: International Universities Press.

Koplowitz, H. (1984). A projection beyond Piaget's formal operations stage: A general systems stage and a unitary stage. In J. L. Commons, F. A. Richards, & C. Armon (Eds.), *Beyond formal operations: Late adolescent and adult cognition development* (pp. 272–295). New York: Praeger.

Kuhn, T. S. (1970). *The structure of scientific revolutions.* (2nd ed.). Chicago: University of Chicago Press. (Original work published 1962)

LaHaye, T. & Phillips, B. (1982). *Anger is a choice.* Grand Rapids, MI: Zonderran.

Lazarus, A. (1981). *The practice of multimodal therapy.* New York: McGraw-Hill.

LeCron, L. (1970). *Self-hypnotism: The technique and its use in daily living.* New York: Signet. (Original work published 1964)

LeShan, L. & Margenau, H. (1982). Einstein's space in Van Gogh's sky. *Physical reality and beyond*. New York: Macmillan.

Levine, S. V. (1979). The role of psychiatry in the phenomenon of cults. *Canadian Journal of Psychiatry, 24*, 593–603.

Lewis, J. M. & Usdin, G. (1982). *Treatment planning in psychiatry*. American Psychiatric Association.

Lowen, A. (1967). *The betrayal of the body*. New York: Macmillan.

Lowen, A. (1972). *Depression and the body*. New York: Coward, McCann & Geoghegan.

Lowen, A. (1975). *Bioenergetics*. New York: Coward, McCann & Geoghegan.

Lowen, A. (1983). *Narcissism: Denial of the true self*. New York: Macmillan.

Lowen, W. (1982). *Dichotomies of the mind: A system science model of the mind and personality*. New York: Wiley Interscience.

Luborsky, L., McLellan, T., Woody, G. E., O'Brien, C. P., & Auerbach, A. (1985). Therapist success and its determinants. *Archives of General Psychiatry, 42*, 602–611.

Marmor, J. (1983). Systems thinking in psychiatry: Some theoretical and clinical implications. *The American Journal of Psychiatry, 140*, 833–838.

Martin, P. A. (1971). Dynamic considerations of the hysterical psychosis. *American Journal of Psychiatry, 128*, 745–748.

Masterson, J. F. (1981). *The narcissistic and borderline disorders*. New York: Brunner/Mazel.

Masterson, J. F. (1985). *The real self: A developmental, self, and object relations approach*. New York: Brunner/Mazel.

May, P. R. A. (1968). *Treatment of schizophrenia: A comparative study of five treatment methods*. New York: Science House.

Melges, F. T. (1982). *Time and the inner future: A temporal approach to psychiatric disorders*. New York: John Wiley & Sons.

Menninger, K. (1973). *Whatever became of sin?* New York: Hawthorne.

Miller, A. (1981). *Prisoners of childhood: The drama of the gifted child and the search for the true self*. New York: Basic Books. (Original work published 1979)

Miller, J. G. & Miller, J. L. (1985). General living systems theory. In H. I. Kaplan & B. J. Sadock (Eds.), *Comprehensive Textbook of Psychiatry, Vol. IV* (pp. 13–24). Baltimore/London: Williams & Wilkins.

Millon, T. (1981). *Disorders of personality, DSM-III: Axis II*. New York: John Wiley & Sons.

Nalimov, V. V. (1982). *Realms of the unconscious: The enchanted frontier*. Philadelphia, PA: ISI Press.

Nardone, D. A. (1986, in press). Collecting and analyzing data: Doing and thinking. In K. Walker, D. Hall, & W. Hurst (Eds.), *Clinical methods*. Butterworth.

Niebuhr, R. (1956). *An interpretation of Christian ethics*. New York: Meridian. (Original work published 1935)

Orne, M. T. (1959). The nature of hypnosis: Artifact and essence. *Journal of Abnormal and Social Psychology, 58*, 277–299.

Pearson, D. J., Rix, K. J. B., & Bentley, S. J. (1983). Food allergy: How much is in the mind? A clinical and psychiatric study of suspect food hypersensitivity. *Lancet, 1*, 1259–1261.

Peck, M. S. (1983). *People of the lie: The hope for healing human evil*. New York: Simon & Schuster.

Perls, F. S. (1969). *Gestalt therapy verbatim*. Lafayette, CA: Real People Press.

Popper, K. R. (1959). *The logic of scientific discovery*. New York: Harper & Row.

Poundstone, W. (1985). *The recursive universe: Cosmic complexity and the limits of scientific knowledge.* Chicago: Contemporary Books, Inc.

Pribram, K. H. (1971). *Languages of the brain.* Monterey, CA: Brooks/Cole.

Prince, M. (1969). *The dissociation of a personality.* New York: Greenwood Press. (Original work published 1906)

Randolph, T. G. (1956). The descriptive features of food addiction: Addictive eating and drinking. *Quarterly Journal for the Study of Alcoholism, 17,* 198–224.

Rhine, J. B. (1937). *New frontiers of the mind.* New York: Farrar & Rhinehart.

Riedl, R. (1984). *Biology of knowledge: The evolutionary basis of reason.* New York: John Wiley & Sons.

Roberts, J. (1974). *The nature of personal reality: A Seth book.* Englewood Cliffs, NJ: Prentice Hall.

Roberts, J. (1976). *The coming of Seth.* New York: Pocket Books. (A Reprint of J. Roberts, *How to develop your esp power.* New York: Frederick Fell, 1966)

Rosnow, R. L. (1983). Von Osten's horse, Hamlet's question, and the mechanistic view of causality: Implications for a post-crisis social psychology. *The Journal of Mind and Behavior, 4,* 319–338.

Rossi, E. (Ed.). (1980). The collected works of Milton H. Erickson, M.D., *Vols. I-IV.* New York: Irvington.

Rothstein, A. (1980). Psychoanalytic paradigms and their narcissistic investment. *Journal of the American Psychoanalytic Association, 28,* 385–395.

Rucker, R. (1982). *Infinity and the mind: The science and philosophy of the infinite.* Boston: Birkhaüser.

Russell, B. (1948). *Human knowledge: Its scope and limits.* New York: Simon & Schuster.

Sarbin, T. R. (1944). The logic of prediction in psychology. *Psychological Review, 51,* 210–228.

Sarbin, T. R. & Coe, W. C. (1972). *Hypnosis: A social psychological analysis of influence communication.* New York: Holt, Rhinehart & Winston.

Schacht, T. & Nathan, P. E. (1977). But is it good for psychologists? Appraisal and status of DSM-III. *American Psychologist, 32,* 1017–1025.

Sheehan, P. W. & Perry, C. W. (1976). *Methodologies of hypnosis: A critical appraisal of contemporary paradigms of hypnosis.* Hillsdale, NJ: Lawrence Erlbaum.

Shenk, L. & Bear, D. (1981). Multiple personality and related dissociative states in patients with temporal lobe epilepsy. *The American Journal of Psychiatry, 138,* 1311–1316.

Simonton, O., Matthew-Simonton, S., & Creighton, J. (1978). *Getting well again: A step-by-step self-help guide to overcoming cancer for patients and their families.* Los Angeles: Martins Press.

Smedes, L. B. (1984). *Forgive and forget: Healing the hurts we don't deserve.* San Francisco, CA: Harper & Row.

Smith, J. R. (1982). Personal responsibility in traumatic stress reaction. *Psychiatric Annals, 12*(11), 1021–1027.

Snedecor, G. W. & Cochran, W. G. (1967). *Statistical methods.* Ames, IA: The Tower State University Press.

Sontag, F. (1977). *Sun Myung Moon and the Unification Church.* Nashville: Abington.

Spanos, N. P. (in press). Hypnotic behavior: A social psychological interpretation of amnesia, analgesia and "trance logic." *The Behavioral and Brain Sciences.*

Sparr, L. & Pankratz, L. D. (1983). Factitious posttraumatic stress disorder. *American Journal of Psychiatry, 140,* 1016–1019.

Spiegel, D. (1984). Multiple personality as a post-traumatic stress disorder. In B. G. Braun (Ed.), Multiple personality. *Psychiatric Clinics of North America, 7*, 101–110.

Spinoza, B. (1951). *The ethics*. New York: Dover. (Original work published 1677)

Spitzer, R. L. & Fleiss, J. L. (1974). A re-analysis of the reliability of psychiatric diagnosis. *British Journal of Psychiatry, 125*, 341–347.

Spitzer, R. L., Fleiss, J. L., & Endicott, J. (1967). Quantification of agreement in psychiatric diagnosis. *Archives of General Psychiatry, 17*, 83–87.

Starr, P. (1982). *The social transformation of American medicine*. New York: Basic Books.

Steiner, C. (1979). The pig parent. *Transactional Analysis Journal, 9*, 26–40.

Stent, G. S. (1975). Limits to the scientific understanding of man. *Science, 187*, 152–1057.

Stern, C. (1980). *The etiology of identity splitting in multiple personality dissociations*. Ann Arbor: Universities Microfilms International.

Strupp, H. H. (1980). Success and failure in time-limited psychotherapy. *Archives of General Psychiatry, 37*, 595–603.

Strupp, H. H. & Binder, J. L. (1984). *Psychotherapy in a new key: A guide to time-limited dynamic psychotherapy*. New York: Basic Books.

Sullivan, H. S. (1953). *The interpersonal theory of psychiatry*. New York: Norton.

Szilard, L. (1929). Uber die Entropieverminderung in einem thermodynamischen system bei eingriffen intelligenter wesen. *Zeitschrift fur Physik, 53*, 840–856. (Summarized in W. Poundstone, 1985, pp. 67–77)

Tart, C. T. (1975). *States of consciousness*. New York: E. P. Dutton.

Tavris, C. (1982). *Anger: The misunderstood emotion*. New York: Simon & Schuster.

Teller, E. (1980). *The pursuit of simplicity*. Malibu, CA: Pepperdine University Press.

Terr, L. (1983). Chowchilla revisited: The effects of psychic trauma four years after a school-bus kidnapping. *American Journal of Psychiatry, 140*, 1543–1550.

Tillich, P. (1951). *Systematic theology* (Vol. I). Chicago: University of Chicago Press.

Tou, J. T. & Gonzalez, R. C. (1974). *Pattern recognition principles*. Reading, MA: Addison-Wesley.

Ullman, M., Krippner, S., & Vaughn, A. (1973). *Dream telepathy*. New York: Macmillan.

Vaillant, G. E. (1984). The disadvantages of DSM-III outweight its advantages. *American Journal of Psychiatry, 141*, 542–545.

Van Putten, T. & May, P. R. (1978). Subjective response as a predictor of outcome in pharmacotherapy. *Archives of General Psychiatry, 35*, 477–480.

Verdi, G. & Piave, F. M. (1861). *La forza del destina*. (Opera)

von Bertalanffy, L. (1968). *General systems theory: Foundations, development, application*. New York: Braziller.

von Bertalanffy, L. (1981). *A systems view of man*. Boulder, CO: Western Press.

WTBS Super Station. Russia Under Attack, in *The world at war*, 1985.

Watkins, J. G. (1960). *General psychotherapy: An outline and study guide*. Springfield, IL: C C Thomas.

Watkins, J. G. (1971). The affect bridge: A hypnoanalytic technique. *International Journal of Clinical and Experimental Hypnosis, 19*, 21–27.

Watkins, J. G. (1978). *The therapeutic self*. New York: Human Sciences Press.

Watkins, J. G. & Watkins, H. H. (1979a). Ego states and hidden observers. *Journal of Altered States of Consciousness, 5*.

Watkins, J. G. & Watkins, H. H. (1979b). The theory and practice of ego state therapy. In H. Grayson (Ed.), *Short-term approaches to psychotherapy*. New York: National Institute for the Psychotherapies and Human Science Press.

Watzlawick, P. (1976). *How real is real?* New York: Random House.

Watzlawick, P., Beavin, J. H., & Jackson, D. D. (1967). *Pragmatics of human communication: A study of interactional patterns, pathologies and paradoxes*. New York: Norton.

Watzlawick, P., Weakland, J., & Fisch, R. (1974). *Change: Principles of problem formation and problem resolution*. New York: Norton.

Weakland, J. (1983). Family therapy with individuals. *Journal of Strategic and Systemic Therapies, 2*(4), 1–9.

Webster's Seventh New Collegiate Dictionary (1963). Springfield, MA: G. & C. Merriam Co.

Weeks, G. R. & L'Abate, L. (1982). *Paradoxical psychotherapy: Theory and technique*. New York: Brunner/Mazel.

Weiss, P. (1967). One plus one does not equal two. In G. Querton, T. Melnechuk, & F. O. Schmit (Eds.), *The neurosciences* (pp. 801–821). New York: Rockfeller University Press.

Weitzenhoffer, A. M. & Hilgard, E. R. (1959). *Stanford hypnotic susceptibility scales forms A and B*. Palo Alto: Consulting Psychologists Press.

Weitzenhoffer, A. M. & Hilgard, E. R. (1959). *Stanford hypnotic susceptibility scales form C*. Palo Alto: Consulting Psychologists Press.

Wender, P. H. & Klein, D. F. (1981). *Mind, mood, and medicine*. New York: Farrar, Straus & Giroux.

Wilber, K. (1983). *Eye to eye: The quest for the new paradigm*. New York: Anchor Press.

Williams, J. B. (1985). The multiaxial system of DSM-III: Where did it come from and where should it go? I. Origins and customs. *Archives of General Psychiatry, 42*, 175–180. II. Empirical studies, innovations, and recommendations. *Archives of General Psychiatry, 42*, 181–186.

Woods, S. C. & Kulkosky, P. J. (1976). Classically conditioned changes of blood glucose level. *Psychosomatic Medicine, 38*, 201–219.

Woollams, S., Brown, B., & Huige, N. (1976). *Transactional analysis in brief*. Ypsilanti, MI: Spectrum Psychological Services.

Yager, J. & Young, R. (1974). Non-hypoglycemia is an epidemic condition. *New England Journal of Medicine, 291*, 907–908.

Yalom, I. D. (1971). A study of encounter group casualties. *Archives of General Psychiatry, 25*, 16–30.

Zimmerman, D. W. (1979). Quantum theory and interbehavioral psychology. *The Psychological Record, 29*, 473–485.

Index